DESIGNED TO MOVE

The Science-Backed Program to Fight Sitting Disease and Enjoy Lifelong Health

Joan Vernikos

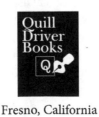

Fresno, California

Published by Quill Driver Books
An imprint of Linden Publishing
2006 South Mary Street, Fresno, California 93721
(559) 233-6633 / (800) 345-4447
QuillDriverBooks.com

Quill Driver Books and Colophon are trademarks of
Linden Publishing, Inc.

ISBN 978-1-61035-271-0

135798642

Printed in the United States of America
on acid-free paper.

Library of Congress Cataloging-in-Publication Data

Names: Vernikos, Joan, author.
Title: Designed to move : the science-backed program to fight sitting
disease
  and enjoy lifelong health / Joan Vernikos.
Description: Fresno, California : Quill Driver Books, 2017. | Includes
  bibliographical references and index.
Identifiers: LCCN 2017001529 | ISBN 9781610352710 (pbk. : alk. paper)
Subjects: LCSH: Exercise--Physiological aspects--Popular works. | Physical
  fitness--Popular works. | Gravity--Physiological effect. | Health--Popular
  works. | Self-care, Health--Popular works.
Classification: LCC RA781 .V46 2017 | DDC 613.7--dc23
LC record available at https://lccn.loc.gov/2017001529

This book is dedicated to the magnificent John Glenn:
hero, astronaut, U.S. senator, and, most of all, a wonderful human being.

Contents

Part One: Astronauts, Aging, and Sitting

Part Two: How to Enjoy Lifelong Health Through Smart and Frequent Movement

Foreword

My good friend, respected colleague, and former boss' boss, Dr. Joan Vernikos will surprise and motivate you to better health through her wonderful book, *Designed to Move*. I've been fortunate to know Joan for more decades than I'd care to acknowledge, dating back to my fledgling laboratory days at the NASA Ames Research Center. Back then, I was a young Stanford medical student working at the center, with ambitions of one day flying in space. Joan oversaw the entire spaceflight life sciences research program. Since the early days of NASA's space program, she has been an iconic pioneer in discovering the ways in which the human body adapts to the weightlessness of space, and then readapts to earth's gravity coming back home.

My wonderful career has allowed me to rocket up into space on five occasions, venture out into the vacuum of space on seven dramatic spacewalks, and later forge my way to the summit of Mount Everest on foot. Resilience and extreme fitness certainly helped me attain those wonderful summits, but science has challenged us all to reconsider the notion of good health. While cardiovascular and strength training certainly have an important role in health and longevity, and were essential in my expeditions in life, are there simple measures that all of us can follow to enjoy true health? Joan makes a very compelling, scientific-but-readable case for *movement*— one that we should all heed.

The older I've gotten, the more it's become apparent that it's not how long we live, but how long we live *well*. *Designed to Move* gives us the solution to improve our health and well-being, motivating us to invigorate our often sedentary, seated lifestyles. Skillfully distilling the medical literature, Joan shows us powerful ways to challenge gravity and both live long and prosper!

You can do this.

Onward and upward,
Scott Parazynski, M.D.
Houston, Texas

Introduction

Throughout my fifty-five years in the space business, I was regularly asked about how we could send humans to live on Mars. How would our ancient genes fare in deep space and on foreign planets? The question is not much different here on Earth. How can we humans, with our ancestral genes, thrive in today's or tomorrow's technology-modified environment?

My research at NASA was devoted to keeping astronauts healthy. Their bodies go through changes as they respond and seek to adapt to living in the microgravity of space. The research revealed unexpected clues to just how crucial gravity is to all of us living here on Earth. Plants need gravity to thrive, as do birds and bees to fly and navigate. Yet we humans generally ignore gravity. Yes, we know it's all around us, but so what? Medical texts never mention it. If asked, we think of gravity as the enemy that drags us down and ages us. But I found that gravity is undoubtedly our friend, if only we would use it.

While I was speaking to audiences of all ages and writing *The G-Connection: Harness Gravity and Reverse Aging* (2004) and later *Sitting Kills, Moving Heals* (2011), new questions came up. I realized that I was sitting—excuse the pun—on a goldmine of information that could literally help millions live healthier, and therefore happier, longer lives in our ever-accelerating modern technology-rich society. Some of these technologies and medical advances help us live longer. But are we healthier? I therefore felt an urgency to share my knowledge and ideas based on new questions and data that may help you adjust and thrive in this fast-moving age. *Designed to Move* summarizes these new concepts in an effective but different way from the traditional pills, diet, and exercise commonly used as the solution to our ills.

Since I wrote *Sitting Kills, Moving Heals*, more information has been published about the hazards of sitting. Mostly this is based on metadata analyses and statistical surveys of existing epidemiological information, all linking our sedentary behavior to most modern disorders. This new evidence on the disastrous consequences of the hours we spend sitting has fueled huge social concern. Reliable research studies are rare. Effective solutions are even harder to find. It seemed obvious to me that the root of this social problem is that we just don't move much any more.

Move is a very interesting word. If you are not moving, you may be taken for dead. Whether verb or noun, this ancient word is loaded with life. It is equivalent to energy. The *Oxford English Dictionary* traces its origins to the ancient French *mouvoir* and the Latin *movere*. It has come to mean a lot of things. Appearing in the fifteenth century in reference to chess, it was later associated with moving furniture or relocating to a house or making a strategic move; it may be as practical as digesting, or having a bowel movement or a racing heart rate. A book, poem, or admirer may be deeply moving, invoking the inner stirrings of emotion. Essentially, moving is defined as a change in position, whether internal, external, or emotional.

Movelessness, then, is what you do when sitting. It involves minimal motion. "He is not moving" is taken to mean someone is not in any form of action, is lifeless, without energy or dead. Considering moving in all its variations is essential to understanding life. Communicating the pivotal role of moving in staying healthy and alive is this book's message.

Designed to Move is for those who want to regain control over their long-term health and well-being with a natural solution. I wrote it to bring you up to speed on the latest research from NASA and the scientific community on the physiological benefits of moving and to offer workable solutions for using gravity, our ever-present friend, to strengthen your body and improve your life. As we struggle to find the best ways to help astronauts explore and live on Mars one day, why not at the same time choose to live well on Earth? This book shows you how.

Part One

Astronauts, Aging, and Sitting

Chapter 1

Gravity Gets You Moving

As we progress through life in today's society, we become more and more sedentary. We call the changes "aging," as if they are natural and unavoidable. It does not have to be that way. Our genes may predispose but how healthy your aging might be is at your disposal. Learning how to live in gravity is what children do as they learn to move in the earliest months and years of life. Relearning how to live in gravity as an adult is what this book is all about. Gravity is more than our friend—it is our lifeline.

In 1964, I was hired by the National Aeronautics and Space Administration (NASA) as a postdoctoral fellow. My job was to help NASA conduct research on stress and how astronauts could cope with the rigors of traveling into outer space and back to Earth. This was three years after the first human (Soviet cosmonaut Yuri Gagarin) had flown into space, an event that prompted U.S. president John F. Kennedy to issue the famous challenge to put a man on the moon by the end of the decade. Though I held a Ph.D. from a highly regarded medical school, I knew nothing about how travel in outer space might affect the human body, and neither did anyone else. In my medical research I had plenty of experience measuring stress in humans under a variety of conditions. My research specialty involved developing new and better ways of measuring the hormone response to stress and discovering how the brain was involved in that response. One thing that seemed clear to NASA and everyone else was that putting humans on top of a rocket and blasting them into space had to be stressful. It was therefore logical that the small team of five scientists who formed the first core of NASA's research group at the Ames Research Center in California should include a person with my background as their stress researcher.

And so it was that I came to have access to the hormone data from samples obtained from astronauts Frank Borman and Jim Lovell before, during, and after the historic fourteen-day Gemini 7 space mission in

1965, the longest manned space flight at that time. Though we found, as we had in previous flights, sizeable increases in stress hormones like cortisol before launch and after landing fourteen days later, this was the first time we had the opportunity to measure stress hormones daily throughout the astronauts' actual stay in space.

You may well imagine my astonishment when the stress hormones, rather than being increased, were in fact reduced during the flight—reduced to well below their normal Earth levels, let alone the increased pre- and postflight levels. After exhausting the possibilities of some sort of error, my conclusion was that living in space without gravity was less stressful (for some, at least*) than living on Earth. Far from being a stress, it was the achievement of a dream.**

Not wanting to lose my job with NASA because of this unexpected result, I quickly had to find some other aspect of space flight to study. Considering that astronauts in space spent their time in microgravity—specifically, about one-millionth of Earth's gravity—it occurred to me that space flight provided us the opportunity to study life in this reduced-gravity environment. Since my previous research had studied stress, I considered the question whether reduced gravity—absurd as it might seem—was itself a stress condition. I decided to turn my research focus to gravity and how it might affect normal physiology. Like most of you, I had learned about gravity at school, about Sir Isaac Newton and falling apples hitting the ground. I knew that gravity was all around us, keeping us from floating away from Earth, but like most people I had simply taken gravity for granted, until the Gemini astronauts' test results forced me to look at it in a new way.

THE MYSTERY OF MICROGRAVITY

As advances in the space program captured headlines and fascinated the public, everyone from physicists to psychics soon came out with theories about what might be expected to occur in microgravity. The ones given scientific credence were based on the hypothesis that a human in space flight must be in a condition of inactivity; any exercise was presumed to be ineffective without working against the force of gravity. The NASA program was therefore heavily focused on this premise.

---

* The original seven astronauts were a very select group who had seen action in Vietnam or Korea and were fulfilling their passion of reaching space.
** It should be noted that results from later flights during ensuing years seemed to at least partially contradict these 1965 findings.

To address the presumed need for resistant exercise, over the years increasingly sophisticated space vehicles were fitted with various forms of exercise equipment, including a variety of treadmills, bicycle ergometers, and stretch-bands, as well as complex, expensive, one-of-a kind resistive exercise devices designed specifically to function in space. Russian cosmonauts are said to have exercised for up to four hours a day on a treadmill, and there are reports of astronauts or cosmonauts who had exercised on treadmills nearly all day. In 1996, the American astronaut Shannon Lucid apparently did so during her 179-day stay on the Russian space station *Mir*. She returned in relatively good condition, as did Sunita Williams, whose goal was to run a marathon on the treadmill on the *International Space Station (ISS)* Expedition 14 in 2006. A Russian cosmonaut who had a falling-out with his crewmates is said to have spent most of his day on the treadmill to avoid having to interact with his crewmates, which of course also meant that others could not use it.

What is interesting is that those who exercised throughout the day, whether incessantly or in short intervals, seemed to have returned to Earth healthier than those who exercised for a stint of two to four hours once a day. Similarly, those who had to perform work outside the spacecraft (extra-vehicular activity, or EVA) seemed to exhibit physiological benefits from this training. Whether their task was to launch a satellite or carry out repairs, they had to work strenuously for almost a day in their special space suits in difficult conditions. However, test results indicated that this work mostly involved the upper body and did not benefit their legs and lower spine. Thus, the popular conclusion was that avoiding inactivity was the key to maintaining good health in space. But, as important as it might be to counteract inactivity in microgravity, I was never quite sure that inactivity was the whole story.

In my early days at NASA, I was asked to write the first "NASA Space Biomedical Research Plan," which was published in 1968. We had very little data to go on at that time. We knew from the Mercury and early Gemini flights, as well as hearsay from the Soviet cosmonauts, that nausea and sometimes vomiting were the first symptoms experienced during space flight and could last up to four days. Astronauts also experienced a relative dehydration that could amount to as much as a 10 percent reduction in plasma volume. This showed up when they returned home as reduced body weight, visibly skinny legs (for which Pete Conrad was famously referred to as "chickenlegs"), and faintness on standing. Once back on Earth, however, the fluid loss recovered very quickly.

In preparing to write that research plan, I asked a handful of colleagues from Stanford University to meet with me for a brainstorming session one Saturday morning in 1966. My goal was to share with them what little I knew and what I could glean from my Gemini stress data, and to see what ideas they might come up with. Bill Dement, a pioneer in sleep research, Julian Davidson, a leader in sex behavior research, Fred Melges, a psychologist who worked on self-image and wondered how astronauts would feel about themselves in an environment that had no up or down, and Gig Levine, who, like me, specialized in aspects of behavior and stress, formed the team. The creative exchange we had that day gave me a totally different perspective on the extraordinary relationship of humans to gravity here on Earth.

Thanks to the ideas shared by these brilliant colleagues, I realized that gravity, being one of the major forces of the universe, provides a source of stimulation here on Earth, depending on our relationship to it. If we do not use it, we might as well be in space.

Gravity is a relatively fixed unidirectional force pulling us downward towards the center of the Earth. This stimulus we feel can be physical, such as providing weight and making our muscles work during activity, but primarily it is sensed through the vestibular system in the inner ear and sensors throughout our body—in the soles of our feet, palms of our hands, and our seat—to give us the sense of direction and acceleration that enable us to relate to our environment as we move. Pilots talk about flying "by the seat of their pants" when they had no navigational equipment and rely on sensing gravity as they are pinned to their seat when taking a sharp turn, "pulling Gs."

Gravity also happens to be our biggest source of fun. This realization brought home to me the concept that whether it be stress or gravity, electrical or magnetic stimulation, or heat or pain that are the stimulus, the response will depend on how we perceive it. Indeed, in the early days of the space race Disney had produced a short film titled *Man in Space* (1955) that was shown in theaters and on television and adapted into the Tomorrowland "Rocket to the Moon" ride at the Disneyland amusement park. There an invisible, automated adjustment of the seats gave visitors sensations intended to simulate the increased Gs of "blastoff," followed by a sense of "weightlessness" upon breaking free of Earth's orbit. In real life, NASA's early Gemini astronauts probably perceived being gravity-free in space as a delight and a fulfillment of dreams, especially when compared to surviving in their previous military life in near-miss missions during the Korean Vietnam war. Cardiologist and astronaut Dr. Drew Gaffney, who flew on the Shuttle SLS-2 mission in 1991, referred to his first moments in space as "an immense sense of freedom," even though he was strapped tightly into his space suit and seat during launch.

SPACE, AGING, AND AN ELDERLY ASTRONAUT

On February 10, 1962—some two years before I came to work at NASA—astronaut John Glenn became the first American to orbit the Earth. It was thirty-five years later, one day in 1997, that an instantly recognizable Senator Glenn walked into my office at NASA headquarters in Washington, D.C. He had long wanted to go back into space, having been denied that opportunity by President Kennedy. The grounds for that presidential decision had to do with the political impact of potentially losing a national hero in case of any mishap or failure of the mission.

Glenn now brought his case before me in my position as NASA's Director of Life Sciences, arguing that there was scientific value to what could be learned from studying older humans in space, not least about what we could learn about aging on Earth. The oldest astronaut who had flown up to that point in time was Story Musgrave at 61 on the shuttle *Columbia* (STS-80) in 1996. Glenn, 77 years old and a politician himself, had been chair of the Senate Committee on Aging. He had been impressed by the various testimonies he had heard about issues of aging: muscle weakness, bone density loss, poor coordination, and slowed reaction time. From his firsthand experience in space, the list of age-related changes he heard described was all too familiar. He referred to a pamphlet[1] I had written on my observations of the similarities between space flight and aging. Unlike most politicians I had met, who relied on information from their staffers, Glenn had done his own extensive reading on the two conditions.

Yet in trying to decide whether it was worth sending Glenn back into space, I realized the similarities he had observed were a far cry from concluding that the two conditions—space and aging—were identical. The next step was to consult with the researchers and director at the National Institute on Aging as well as with scientists throughout the community. Ultimately, there seemed no reason why he should not go back into space. If his response to space now was different than those of his other six young crewmates, most would have said, "I told you so. What did you expect?"

7

If, on the other hand, health rather than age was the critical factor, Glenn's response would be no different than the other six astronauts. We took into account Glenn's excellent physical condition and recommended he should fly at the ripe age of 78. The shuttle *Discovery* was launched in November 1998 for a nine-day mission, STS-98. The rest is history. Senator Glenn set the bar for the realization that older astronauts, indeed older humans, could and should be allowed to fly if they had the special skills required.

Naturally all of us scientists were extremely keen to know how he would fare, even though we had every pre-flight indication that he was in fine condition. To our relief, his physiological responses during flight were identical to five of his six crewmates. In fact, one 35-year-old was the outlier and fared less well—to which I could only say, "It happens." Glenn's recovery after returning to Earth, which had been something that concerned me, was also quite normal. Clearly what mattered was not a question of age, but a question of his determination to return to space, of his health status and his resilience, features we have come to recognize as healthy aging.

Bed rest simulates gravity deprivation

During the many years between my first studies at NASA and Senator Glenn's return to space, I had, of course, been continuing to probe for answers about how to maintain health when exposed to microgravity. The evidence from astronauts returning from space pointed to inactivity being only part of the story, and my task was to find out the rest of the story.

This was easier said than done, however, because of certain built-in constraints on how NASA could design studies and collect data. In an ideal world, I might have wished to conduct an experiment with some astronauts exercising in space and others not exercising. For ethical reasons, this was not possible, since we believed exercise was essential to counteract the changes that were consistently observed from microgravity exposure. Assigning an astronaut to remain inactive in space would have been unacceptably harmful. To this day, therefore, all data of the persistent and progressive changes reported in space throughout the 50-plus years of humans in space have been in astronauts who did some form of exercise, whether prescribed or on their own initiative.

How, then, could I find a way to compare the effects of gravity deprivation among people who exercised and people who didn't? Coming at

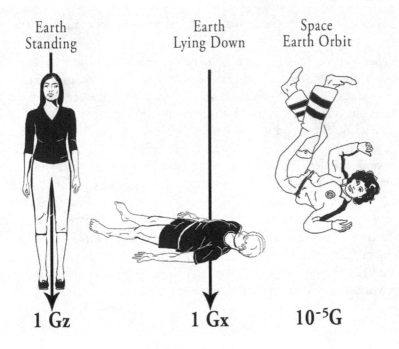

Earth Standing — 1 Gz

Earth Lying Down — 1 Gx

Space Earth Orbit — $10^{-5}G$

**Figure 1. Gravity force and direction (z or x vector) in
relation to the human body.**

research from the perspective that the body has a head, I asked myself what would happen if people on Earth were deprived of gravity's pull from the head downward, as happens when we lie down. From this idea came bed-rest studies, experiments with volunteers lying in bed continuously for days.

A colleague, Dr. John Greenleaf at the Ames Research Center, who specialized in metabolism, had used this technique, as had a few of us at the invitation of Dr. Pauline Beery-Mack, nutrition researcher at Texas Woman's University. By the mid-1970s, I also knew that bed rest, specifically 6-degree, head-down bed rest (HDBR), had been tested by Russian scientists after returning cosmonauts commented that they slept better when back on Earth if the foot of the bed was raised by about 15 inches. This position counteracted the odd post-flight sensation that they were sliding off the foot of their horizontal bed, which made it hard for them to fall asleep—but for scientists, it provided a fruitful line of research. It made sense to me. I introduced this technique in the U.S. and found that it did indeed induce changes similar to those of living without gravity in space.

HDBR soon became the universal model of choice for studying the effects of spaceflight.

The next logical step after simulating the effects of gravity deprivation was to examine the possibility of recovery. It is easy to observe that astronauts in space and HDBR volunteers recover after they return from space or get out of bed respectively, and that, in contrast, people don't "recover" from aging. But could it be possible that the changes we experience as we age are due to lifestyle rather than chronological age? I put the concept forward in *Inactivity: Its Physiology*, a book Hal Sandler and I had edited in 1986[2], and later in *The G-Connection: Harness Gravity and Reverse Aging* in 2004[3]. What we had learned about gravity brought a totally different way of viewing the process of aging and the idea that we could actively influence how we age. It could mean that age-related changes like those Senator Glenn learned about as chair of the Senate Committee on Aging could be delayed and even reversed by adjusting the rate of physical and mental deterioration through lifestyle changes.

Gravity deprivation

Astronauts and bed-rest studies showed us something crucial: They uncovered the unsuspected medical connections between the health hazards of living in microgravity in space, on the one hand, and the chronic diseases that accompany aging on the other. Yet why would reducing gravity in space or bed rest produce similar changes? Then in 2000, I happened to be on a panel with Dr. Alexandre Kalachi, who headed the Aging Section at the World Health Organization (WHO). He showed a chart of how health and physiological functions change during the aging process that got me thinking.

Physiological changes in highly fit astronauts in the near-zero gravity of space, or those caused in healthy men and women by continuous sitting or lying in bed, are similar to those in the elderly. These conditions, which afford negligible use of gravity both in space and here on Earth, produce aging changes and accelerate the aging process. The common denominator of these changes, whether on Earth or in space, is gravity deprivation of one form or another: near-zero gravity in space, reduced influence of gravity when lying down, reduced sensing of gravity or minimal use of gravity here on Earth—in spite of being constantly surrounded by gravity—by habitual prolonged sitting and immobility.

Reduced Gz	Reduced Influence of Sensing Gz	Reduced Use of Gz
Space		
	Newborn babies	
	Water immersion	
	Bed rest and head-down bed rest	
	Illness	
	Injury	
	Surgery	
	Spinal cord injury	
	Children with congenital defects	
		Sitting
		Aging

Table 1. The Gravity Deprivation Syndrome. Conditions that result in common changes resulting from gravity deprivation because of reduced exposure, sensing, or use of gravity. (Gz refers to the head-to-toe vector in which we experience gravity when we stand.)

Here is one example of a gravity deprivation effect that may not be very obvious. The response to one's sense of survival, the ability to spontaneously flee from real or perceived danger on Earth, depends on the readiness of physical responsiveness, the ability of nerves and muscles to react rapidly. This state of preparation is achieved only by continuous, repetitive gravity-using movement. Minimal gravity in space, as was found in later measurements in astronauts during the Skylab and Shuttle missions, is inadequate to maintain such optimal physical responsiveness. In other words, gravity deprivation leads to reduced reaction time.

Other conditions that can result in gravity deprivation include bed rest or immobilization resulting from illness where the illness may be aggravated and recovery delayed, surgery that prevents mobility, congenital damage such as cerebral palsy that compromises the ability to respond normally to gravity, or conditions where the ability to sense gravity has been reduced such as in spinal cord injury. Table 2 lists the main gravity deprivation conditions.

Some obvious consequences of gravity deprivation include reduced endurance, weaker muscles and bones, impaired balance and coordination, back pain, poor sleep with an increased need to urinate at night, disturbed blood pressure regulation, and reduced immune defenses that may result in increased vulnerability to infection.

Table 2 lists more changes that result from spending time in space or bed rest or as we age. These changes are the same as those expected from any condition of gravity deprivation.

In Space or Head-Down Bed Rest (HDBR)	Earth with Age
Decreased plasma volume by 10–20% in 7–180 days	Decreased plasma volume by 0.5–1% per decade
Decreased aerobic capacity by 10–20% in 4–180 days	Decreased aerobic capacity by 10% per decade
Decreased heart stroke volume/ decreased cardiac output	Decreased heart stroke volume/ decreased cardiac output
Decreased heart muscle mass by 1%/cardiomyopathy (unknown)	Decreased heart muscle mass by 1% per year/scarring
Decreased sensitivity of baroreflex	Decreased sensitivity of baroreflex
Arterial stiffness	Arterial stiffness
Blood vessel loss of endothelium lining and nitric oxide	Blood vessel lose of endothelium lining and nitric oxide
Decreased brain blood flow/ decreased cerebral oxygenation	Decreased brain blood flow/ decreased cerebral oxygenation
Increased orthostatic hypotension post-flight or HDBR	Increased orthostatic hypotension on standing up
Decreased muscle mass by 1% per month in legs/spine	Reduced muscle mass by 1% per year

Table 2. Comparison of physiological changes in microgravity or head-down bed rest (HDBR) and aging on Earth. (Table continues on pp. 13–14.)
Reproduced with permission of the Encyclopedia of Bioastronautics, *Springer, 2016.*

In Space or Head-Down Bed Rest (HDBR)	Earth with Age
Decreased muscle protein synthesis within hours	Decreased muscle protein synthesis
Decreased sensitivity to insulin	Decreased sensitivity to insulin/ prediabetic/diabetes
Decreased proportional muscle strength	Decreased proportional muscle strength
Flabby muscles	Flabby muscles
Decreased force/explosive power	Decreased force/explosive power
Slower movement and reaction time	Slower movement and reaction time
Increased body fat replaces muscle	Increased body fat replaces muscle
Increased body fat infiltrates liver in HDBR	Increased body fat infiltrates liver
Decreased lower body bone density by up to 5% per month/ loss of calcium in legs and spine/ osteoporosis	Decreased bone density by 1% per year/loss of calcium in legs, spine, wrists
Risk of bone fracture/kidney stones	Risk of bone fracture/kidney stones
Decreased collagen/aching joints	Decreased collagen/aching joints
Decreased vitamin D3	Decreased vitamin D3
Decreased growth hormone and decreased growth hormone response to exercise	Decreased growth hormone and decreased growth hormone response to exercise
Decreased testosterone	Decreased testosterone
Skin loss of endothelium and nitric oxide	Skin loss of endothelium and nitric oxide
Decreased telomeres and telomerase	Decreased telomeres and telomerase
Cumulative sleep loss	Cumulative sleep loss

Table 2 (cont.) Comparison of physiological changes in microgravity or head-down bed rest (HDBR) and aging on Earth.

In Space or Head-Down Bed Rest (HDBR)	Earth with Age
Circadian dysrhythmia	Circadian dysrhythmia
Brain shrinkage/unknown	Brain shrinkage
Decreased gastric motility/gut transit time/absorption	Decreased gastric motility/gut transit time/absorption
Possible urinary incontinence in women post-flight	Urinary incontinence
Tender soles on walking	Tender soles on getting out of bed
Poor balance/loss of sense of falling post-flight	Poor balance/loss of sense of falling
Poor coordination	Poor coordination/falls
Decreased thirst/hearing/taste	Decreased thirst/hearing loss/taste loss
Vision problems	Vision problems
Increased inflammation and oxidative stress	Increased inflammation and oxidative stress
Immunosuppresion	Immunosuppresion
Viral reactivation/increased bacterial growth in vitro	Viral reactivation/sensitivity to infection
Resistance to antibiotics in vitro	Resistance to antibiotics
Decreased wound healing	Decreased wound healing

Table 2 (cont.) Comparison of physiological changes in microgravity or head-down bed rest (HDBR) and aging on Earth.

More common disorders are discovered every day as the research in space continues.

Astronauts returning from space have to relearn how to use gravity after they land back on Earth in order to recover. As Table 2 indicates, the same is true for those lying in bed for a long time, whether bed-rest volunteers or anyone after surgery or illness, or even after a few days of the flu when they stand up again and try to walk around. A baby born from the relative weightlessness of the womb has to learn how to move for the first time in

Earth's gravity and use it to guide its development to be best adapted to life on Earth. Children growing up make the best and fullest use of G.

Although we are surrounded by gravity on Earth, we can nevertheless deprive ourselves of its benefits. An astronaut in space, a baby, someone lying in bed or as most of us, younger or older, sit, we experience different degrees on this continuum of gravity deprivation by sharing the same characteristic disorders and disabilities. The baby cannot hold its head up or walk until it begins to become adapted to gravity. The astronaut's mobility, a bedridden patient in hospital or an older person in a nursing home who can hardly stand, all experience various degrees of gravity deprivation.

Returning astronauts and bed-rest volunteers are in exactly the same predicament with regard to gravity deprivation. Once back on Earth after a couple of weeks in space, or up and about after a month in bed, they recover. We have learned at NASA that all of the changes astronauts undergo are reversible when gravity-using movement is re-introduced upon their return to Earth. However, the longer an astronaut has remained in space, the harder and slower is the recovery. It is not known at this point, with no more than a maximum of one year spent in space, whether and when the point of no return might be reached, when the changes may become irreversible, just as they are in the late stages of aging. So far, indications are that the debilitating health effects of near-zero gravity would continue their downward trend. This knowledge of recovery matters to us all because we have presumed that we do not recover from aging. However, the research suggests that recovery, or at least delaying the rate of aging, should be possible by making the effort to change sedentary habits and lifestyles.

Kalachi pointed out that from age 20, when physiological development is believed to peak, the gradual deterioration in health from aging reaches a point at about age 80 when it hits a risk zone that implies increased danger of debilitating fractures, disease, frailty, compromised independence, and death. We now know that changes like those recognized as aging are not only similar but accelerated in space as well as during prolonged bed rest and are related to living in reduced gravity or not making adequate use of gravity. In the last seven years, it has been increasingly recognized that these changes are also accelerated by sedentary lifestyles which are common among the elderly. Based on those similarities it stands to reason that excessive sedentariness might accelerate the downhill slope and reach the risk zone earlier than expected. Current observations of evidence of accelerated incidence of metabolic and cardiovascular disease, such as

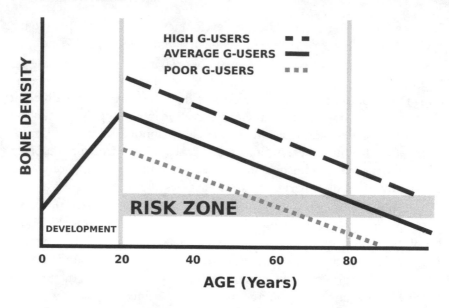

**Figure 2. Hypothetical bone density changes as a function of age.
(Adapted and used with permission from Alexandre Kalachi, WHO.)**

diabetes or stroke in children, have been related to increased sedentary behavior from an early age well below the average risk zone of 80. It would then stand to reason that those that live healthy and active lives to 80 and beyond have done so by remaining active, both physically and cognitively, making greater and more frequent use of gravity. This implies that such greater use of gravity-related moving, such as standing up, often underlie their extended good health habits.

Thinking of gravity like an astronaut gets you moving. Here on Earth the consequences of too much sitting are reversed—regardless of age—when we stand up and move about. We cannot help but use gravity effectively whenever we move. A baby learns to stand and walk by challenging gravity, just as someone who has been bedridden does, as long as they start with a basically healthy body. Gravity is responsible for our sense of weight, direction, acceleration, the change in posture signal, balance, and coordination. Effective gravity-using movement involves frequent changes in all of these aspects, throughout the day, every day. Though these movements are absent in space, we on Earth may enjoy gravity's benefits abundantly. It's merely a matter of choosing to make them part of our daily habits. This book will help you to make that choice.

Chapter 2

The Problem: Prolonged, Uninterrupted Sitting

On average, humans live twenty-five years longer than we did a hundred years ago. The average lifespan was 55 then and is 82 now. But we are not living healthier.

While death from many diseases, including heart disease, cancer, and diabetes, has declined, the incidence of these has increased overall. There are more and more people living with illness now than there used to be. The number of adults with these diseases has increased from 9 to 30 percent in just the last ten years. Plus, on average, we are fatter. In 20- to 74-year-olds, the rate of obesity rose from 25 to 35 percent between 1980 and 2010 alone. Obesity is a major risk factor for a variety of chronic diseases. For example, statistics would tell you that about half of us have neck or back pain at some time. Our well-being is suffering too: The number of Americans reporting challenges from depression and anxiety has steadily increased over the past half century.

What has changed during this period is our lifestyle. We sit too much both at home and at work. Technological and industrial creativity has made our lives easier. But the impact of greatly increased and prolonged sitting on health, productivity, and cost has been disastrous. The 2016 World Health Organization-supported global study headed by professor Ulf Ekelund warns that "increasing inactivity" now costs the world $67.5 billion and 5 million lives a year[4].

WHEN DID WE START SITTING SO MUCH?

Though we have the same genes, our lifestyle has steadily changed from the time humans first started walking about on Earth. Early humans' lives revolved primarily around survival, building tools to construct a shelter for the family, and hunting down sources of water and food. When they sat, it was on the ground, cross-legged, kneeling, or squatting. In ancient Egypt,

Greece, and Rome, benches and stools were the first ordinary seats available until approximately the sixteenth century. A few chairs were made of wood, ebony, or marble, heavily carved, ornate, often gilded. These were symbols of wealth or rank, used as thrones for rulers and ecclesiastical purposes—hence the name *cathedra* (from the Greek *kathedra*, which means sitting on a platform), the seat of a cardinal or bishop. Chairs supported with cross bars by attendants or slaves were also used for transportation of noblemen. The chair is still extensively used as a symbol of authority and privilege. Earlier versions were low with short legs; as the length of the legs increased in more modern times, less effort was required to lower oneself and sit. By the seventeenth century, chairs became common throughout the Western world. By 1818, Lambert Hitchcock in the United States began manufacturing "chairs for the people," making and shipping chair parts for assembly. However, in less developed countries to this day squatting is still the favored method of sitting.

Along with squatting, kneeling is a common position used by the Japanese, many of whom still sleep on floor tatamis in lieu of beds. The multiple times they need to stand up from these positions during a day keeps them healthy. In the early twentieth century, a group of Okinawans were enticed to move to Brazil. In doing this, they adopted the dietary habits of their new home along with Western conveniences such as sitting in chairs and sleeping in beds. In spite of sharing the same genes, data from 100,000 Okinawans showed that their life expectancy was shortened by seventeen years compared to their family relatives who stayed back home. Even in Okinawa, those under 50 who grew up with fast-food outlets surrounding the U.S. military bases now have Japan's highest rates of obesity, heart disease, and premature death. As Western chairs and beds flooded Japan, the level of diabetes has flourished.

One can almost predict the physical mobility of a society by the extent of squatting, kneeling, or floor-sitting habits of its population.

SITTING AT HOME AND SITTING AT THE OFFICE

Human creativity, nurtured by two world wars and the "space race" of the mid-twentieth century, led to the design of machines and appliances developed under the guise of "making our life easier." But these devices gradually robbed us of the many healthy movements we were previously doing. As women entered the workplace, machines were designed that could help make housework easier and faster. The vacuum cleaner meant we did not need to clean and dust every day as our grandparents used to do. The refrigerator and freezer did away with daily walks to the store to shop for perishables. Foods are now precooked and prepackaged, or else we rely on the pizza man to home-deliver dinner. How often do you eat pizza? The washing machine did the hard work of washing for us and the drier replaced the need to hang up the clothes to dry. Now many areas have even outlawed hanging clothes out to dry on the basis of aesthetics.

The motor car—once only for the privileged few and driven by a chauffeur—can now be bought by almost everyone, so we walk less. Then came portable communications products that did not require getting up to answer the phone, and home entertainment systems that encouraged more sitting by eliminating the need to get up to change the TV channel. Pretty soon we shall just speak instructions to the TV. We went to the movies; now the movies come to us through a DVD or the Internet. We wrote letters and went out to post them. Now we write emails or text messages. Electronics are in our hand, news programs are on the Internet, and groceries or other needs can be home-delivered. Yes, progress has been amazing and miraculous. Yet with all these communication devices we are lonely. Our one-on-one physical interactions have dwindled. We may get depressed. There are even plans afoot to offer "loneliness" care to the public. It is as if some devious James Bond movie character contrived to push us back firmly into our chair. We sit more and move less—not just our legs but our entire body, even our faces. When was the last time you shook hands with someone? Or stood up every time a teacher came and left the classroom?

We move less today than at any time in human history. Modern comforts, conveniences, and forms of electronic entertainment deprive us of the simple everyday movement of our recent ancestors. We have no need to move the way we used to. In fact, modern conveniences have robbed people of the many opportunities for movement they once spontaneously encountered by simply going about their lives.

The office is no better. Work for most of us entails sitting in a cubicle in front of a computer all day, or it involves driving a long commute in a car. Until the 1990s, working in an office meant walking from one room to another to speak to colleagues. We used a dial-up phone, exercising our index finger. Today we use email or text messaging; we cannot detach ourselves from social media or smartphones.

Americans now spend an average of 13 hours per week on the internet, while TV time has actually *increased* to 34 hours per week, despite nearly half of us admitting that we watch too much TV. In the office we've almost completely stopped moving. There is no need; we even mindlessly munch on some "lunch" while "working."

We sit during commutes. Mechanized commuting began with the Industrial Revolution in the mid-1800s. Previously, people walked to work. By the turn of this century, we spent more and more time commuting on a train or bus. Today, almost everyone who works drives their own car. We fly long distances in airplanes. Just sitting on a long flight may result in blood clots in leg veins—venous thrombosis—and painful thrombophlebitis, or death from pulmonary embolism. Manual labor has changed as well. Farmers now ride on sophisticated equipment. Agriculture uses tractors, plows, sophisticated sprayers, and harvesting machines. Even a sport like golf has fallen victim to the modern convenience of a golf cart.

Nursing homes should be labeled national sitting centers or pre-death centers. They cannot help it. It's a matter of staff requirements, I've been told. They have optional physical therapy once a day but most residents sit the rest of the time. There are many dreadful nursing homes but also some lovely ones. Last time I visited our best local center I met this beautiful lady in the lobby and stretched out my hand to introduce myself. She stared down at it with a perplexed "What do I do now?" look. When was the last time she had shaken hands with someone, I asked? Children at school are instructed to sit still most of the day. Office workers are expected to sit in front of their computer or at meetings all day. The hours of sitting add up. It comes down to making the most of the time we have, because today it's all about money.

DISCOVERING THE FOUNDATION OF HEALTH

Americans have struggled in recent decades to exercise more and eat less, but one thing hasn't changed: We spend hour after hour every day virtually immobile in our chairs or cars, and we're heavier, sicker, and more tired as a result. The way we live is killing us and we can't seem to stop it. We seem to have had the choice of either sitting or exercising, with nothing—like routine daily movement—in between.

Other cultures have much to teach us. French women, for instance, manage to remain active and slim. Though they are not big fans of the gym, they certainly walk a lot, mostly by simply going about their business of daily living. They also frequently ride bicycles. Bicycles that you may rent and drop off at your destination can be found everywhere.

Fortunately, these are beginning to appear in U.S. cities like San Francisco and Washington, DC. You do not usually see Parisians going for a jog in the park unless they are training for something. However, afternoon strolls to meet friends or get their baguette are common. They go up and down the stairs in the metro and, often, walk up six flights of stairs just to reach the apartment door. We now have elevators in our private homes just to go up one floor! Parisian women are more likely to stay healthy and nimble by doing simple household chores like vacuuming, mopping, and active cleaning, or even taking a dance class, just for the fun of it. Equally, they are fond of going for a walk around the marketplace or at the local square, to meet friends and socialize after an afternoon nap, or they take a short stroll after a late dinner to aid digestion.

In America, our big problem comes from not moving enough as we go about our daily lives. Such smart moving is needed to keep the body tuned and oiled, ready to respond as needed. Its absence makes us heavy, stiff, and rusty. Simple everyday moving is the foundation of health. It's what keeps us alive, resilient, and feeling good. It is very different from working out at the gym.

Alongside the growing popularity of the chair, medical techniques changed in Victorian times to favor practices such as bloodletting and confinement to bed as treatment for almost any disorder. The more affluent people were the more likely they were to be put to bed. The less affluent had to get up and go to work; they probably did themselves a favor. The longer people stayed in bed the weaker they grew, until they became total invalids. They were likely to faint when they tried to stand up, which in turn was promptly treated with more bed rest and so on. The prescription was to "get off one's feet" and "take it easy," advice that can be heard to this day, especially when some new appliance is introduced to replace spontaneous movement.

In the workplace, the Industrial Revolution of the eighteenth century led to long hours of sitting at a job or long hours of standing still at the assembly line or in a retail store. If you were a clerk in Dickensian London, you stood at a high desk or leaned on a high stool. The invention of the electric bulb added the new dimension of shift work. This contributed to poorer health by disrupting natural biological rhythms, thereby reducing adequate sleep. And earlier family practices of sitting down to meals gradually disappeared as everyone in the family either worked or went to school.

Dreadful as World War I was, the cruel imperative to get wounded soldiers out of bed and back to the front line revealed a crucial physiological truth—that the longer they stayed in bed the worse they got. Joseph Pilates was a significant contributor in developing ways of getting these soldiers battle-ready again and, whether he knew it or not at the time, he contributed to revolutionizing medical practices. Today's Pilates classes, which bear limited resemblance to the original methods, are popular for strengthening the body core muscles. World War II reinforced the evidence that whether it was shrapnel injury, amputation, bleeding, or an infection, the act of lying in bed or being immobilized some other way made things worse in all cases. Postwar research on various medical disorders invariably was carried out using patients who were chosen for study of some condition presumably thought to be unrelated to what they were in bed for. For example, persons with a thyroid condition might be used to study the effect of a drug for a cardiovascular disease. Bedridden paraplegics of the first half of the last century would have been amazed at the sports feats of those paralyzed by spinal cord injury today, racing cross-country in their wheelchairs or skiing in special seats.

It was "space race" era research—studying astronauts in space and volunteers in bed rest—that produced the first scientific evidence in healthy volunteers for the fundamental need to move. These studies particularly emphasized the importance of getting people out of bed and ambulatory as soon as possible. It took a while for this knowledge to sink into the practicing physician's conscience. Eventually, this realization led to changing medical attitudes toward treating the injured and the sick and getting people out of bed after surgery. Financial incentives for insurance companies based on these new findings were not far behind, as the opportunity presented itself for larger financial gains by dramatically shortening hospital stays or doing away with them completely by treating the sick as outpatients.

Sustaining a lifetime of well-being largely depends on how well you adjust to the changing conditions in the world around you. Progress and change are unavoidable. They come with each discovery—the first crafted tools, the wheel, the lightbulb, harnessing fossil products, the automobile, the airplane, drones, the rocket, satellites, or humans in space. Change happens and we need to adapt to it, focusing on the benefits as well as the detriments.

But what have we lost because of this? What has been taken away now that we sit so much? Today we sit more and move less, not just our legs but our entire body. When we try to make up for it, we forget the little things, the small movements—brushing our teeth, smiling, touching, winking. Every little bit counts.

MODERN SEDENTARY LIFESTYLES UNDERMINE OUR HEALTH

What's wrong with sitting? It's certainly true that sitting down for brief periods can help us recover from heavy exertions, like working in the fields, construction, road-building, or training for a marathon run. But nowadays, for most of us, our lifestyles cause us to sit much more than we move around. Our bodies are simply not built for such a sedentary existence.

Right now as you read this you are probably sitting down. The longer you sit the more disturbed your body becomes, though you may not notice it at first. Your body is probably counting the minutes till you move again. It is *designed* to move.

If you took an X-ray of yourself, you would find hundreds of bones, joints, ligaments, and muscles whose purpose is to help you move and do whatever you feel like doing, from plain standing up to playing some exotic sport to challenging yourself as an acrobat performer on the Cirque du Soleil. Moving helps your blood to circulate. Yes, it can do this without your moving, but not for long and not very well. Your lymph glands and lymphatic system—so important for our immune defenses and for disposing of toxins—would not drain without movement. Your skin, the largest organ in your body, is elastic and is designed to stretch with every move you make. If you do not move, it will sag.

If you do not move—and sitting or lying in bed are the most common examples of not moving—your spine's discs, which support your body both when it's upright and when you bend and move around, would collapse on each other. A typical way of sitting is with a slumped back and curved shoulders. Take a look at any teenager curved over a texting device for hours on end. Their spine depends on movement and play during development to grow strong and straight. They may grow up permanently stooped in adulthood. I watch a group of women taking their daily walk every lunchtime. Much as I admire them for being out there walking, I can't help but observe that they are all stooped, watching their feet. Stooping puts an uneven strain on muscles and ligaments that stretch to accommodate your body's curved position. It is little wonder that almost everyone suffers from back or neck pain at some point in their life.

When I recently spoke to the Ohio Physical Therapists Association, I was surprised to hear that 80 percent of their clients come in for neck and back pain problems. The rest come for pain of arms, legs, feet, and hands. If you don't move, pain will get you soon enough.

When you stoop forward, you do not fully expand your lungs. They may collapse from undue chest pressure when they have less space to expand when you breathe. That is a problem because less oxygen is circulating through your lungs to carry to other parts of your body. Around the skeleton are the muscles, arteries, and veins, soft tissue that become compressed by sitting; this compression may decrease blood supply to your limbs and may block nerves, which could cause you to feel numbness. The veins in your legs are also compressed, leading to swelling, not only from stooping but also, depending on how you sit, by shutting off circulation to and from the legs at the hip and knee junction. This is made worse if you are pregnant or have some extra fat in your abdomen. And did you know that this sluggish circulation in your legs and lower body affects your brain as it becomes deprived of blood flow and oxygen just when you use it most, when you sit down to work. So, sitting will affect your concentration level as everything your blood flow brings to the brain, such as oxygen and glucose, falls.

Prolonged sitting also affects your metabolism. It leads to inhibition of *lipoprotein lipase*, a special enzyme in the walls of capillaries that breaks down fats in the blood. When you sit, you do not burn fat nearly as well as when you move around. So, something like the sitting that we do all the time has the power to change our health.

The solution is simple and intuitive. When you have no choice but to sit, try switching the slouch for a straighter spine. Better still, set a reminder to yourself to reverse these changes by standing up to regain power. Mostly gain an appreciation that bodies are built for motion, not stillness. In fact, treat your body now. Stand up and stretch. Your body will thank you later.

WHAT DOES SITTING TAKE AWAY?

The obvious answer is that, apart from initially collapsing in your chair, you are not moving. But most peoples' response to the question is that you are inactive, which means that you are not exercising. The other response is that you are not standing.

Exercise has become the antidote to all our ills: the harder the better. Look around you at the proliferation of fitness magazines, exercise programs in the work place, and the proliferation of gyms with "free" membership—paid by your insurance company. Yet most people who begin an exercising program give up. They quit the gym, or they go to the gym but spend most of their time sitting and socializing, which has its own merits but would not be considered exercise. The actual national membership in gyms is 17 percent, of which only about 7 percent are considered active members. Health associations and government guidelines encourage you to exercise, but even die-hard exercisers are not counteracting the effects of sitting the rest of the time.

I heard this argument in the case of astronauts. What does being in space take away? Since astronauts find themselves being relatively inactive because of the almost weightless condition that they find themselves in, some argue it must be exercise. Though exercise helps astronauts with endurance and strength, it does not prevent all the other negative changes observed in space which are similar to but more intense than those caused by sitting too much. What is worse in space is that even if you exercise hard once a day you are still in microgravity the rest of the time. On the ground, when you stop exercising, you are at least in Earth's gravity (1G), even if its influence is reduced when you are sitting. It appeared to me that there was more to this issue in space than just exercise, of which the astronauts get plenty.

So we know a lot about what space does to the body, but what does sitting take away? Well, if you are sitting, you must be inactive. Therefore, it would seem you must need exercise to counteract the effects of sitting. However, even those who exercise regularly show the same problems when they sit. Actually, the research is now showing that exercising at the gym once a day *does not* counteract the effects of sitting for a great part of the rest of the day. Once-a-day exercise does not seem to substitute for all-day spontaneous moving (of the type our pre-industrial ancestors engaged in), and it seems that the body needs to be doing something all day long. As Dorothy Dunlap of Northwestern University put it, "Being sedentary is not a synonym for inadequate physical activity."[5]

While sitting leads to weight gain, spontaneous smart moving that interrupts your sitting leads to weight loss. Dr. James Levine at the Mayo Clinic was the first to raise the importance of fat metabolism changes during sitting. Inactivity as a result of lying in bed also inhibits the appetite-suppressing hormone leptin, thus contributing to weight gain.[6] Studies by Levine[6] as well as Marc Hamilton at the University of Missouri and his colleagues[7,8] have shown that sitting dramatically suppresses the enzyme lipoprotein lipase that gets fat out of the blood stream and into muscle for use during moving. This suppression during sitting leaves excess fat in the blood where it increases the risk of heart disease. If unused, this fat can be stored in the body, in muscle, bone, even the liver and kidney. Smart moving, particularly low level spontaneous activity such as standing up and moving about all day, appears to be the best way to keep lipoprotein lipase in good working order. Exercise and moving about do different things in different ways.

HEALTH IS NOT THE SAME AS FITNESS

What does fitness mean to you? Fitness means different things to different people, depending on what your goals are. Are you trying to lose some weight, get ready for that slinky bathing suit, get up a flight of stairs without huffing, or merely get out of bed painlessly in the morning?

Health and fitness are often used interchangeably but they are not the same, any more than moving all day is the same as exercising once a day. They do different things and act in different ways. The research shows us that exercise is required for strength and endurance, whereas frequent movement is the foundation of health. It provides the continuous healthy physiological baseline on which you may add strength and endurance with exercise. Both are needed but are different in the way they act and complement each other. Exercise and smart moving differ in significant ways:

- Exercise increases oxygen consumption and burns calories to generate energy by contracting muscles and generating heat.

- The effectiveness of moving relies primarily on using gravity. Standing up barely burns any calories though it raises your heart rate and blood pressure, especially if you have not stood up for a while.

- Smart moving requires cognitive, emotional, and physical interaction. Exercise is mostly sterile, whereas smart moving involves a purpose. It is a mindful interaction with nature, the environment, other senses, people, pets, or even turning a job into fun.

- Exercise is mostly high intensity and relies on sugar for fuel, whereas smart moving is low intensity, using body fat for fuel. The calories generated from burning fat are an added bonus.

In fact, my own research showed that after lying in bed continuously for four days, standing up was even more effective than walking in maintaining blood pressure regulation, blood volume, and stamina.[9]

The results showed that the benefits came not from how long one stood up, but how many *times* one stood up from a lying-down position—a minimum of 16 times a day was needed (or an estimated 32 to 36 times per day from a seated position). Standing up every 20 to 30 minutes throughout the day seemed to be the most effective solution, one which I put to good use in various studies. After measuring the time course of various parameters such as plasma volume, heart rate, blood pressure, circulating cortisol, ACTH, plasma rennin, catecholamines, vasopressin, etc., in response to lying down or standing up, we found that the maximum changes occur in the first 20 minutes. As expected, the measurements improved when standing up and worsened when lying down, though these changes continue at a slower rate if the posture is maintained. You hear today the 20-minute standing up recommendation to break up sitting as generally accepted. It seems a safe guess, though an actual study of posture change from sitting was never done.

The mere act of standing up does not burn too many calories, probably no more than 12. So the value of standing up did not appear to be a matter of calories burned or energy generated. Rather, the change in posture triggers the brain balance and the vestibular systems, and causes redistribution of blood throughout the body. This in turn stimulates blood pressure sensors in the heart and neck to maintain blood supply to the brain as you stand. Ideally, these actions should be applied regularly throughout the day, every day, including weekends. So get up on your feet! Changing posture as frequently as you can throughout the day is a break worth taking.

Unfortunately, it does not seem that you can make up for the negative health impact of endless hours of inactivity caused by sitting by dashing to the gym for some exercise. In fact, only difficult maximal exercise seems to be effective at counteracting extensive sitting. In a study we did with my colleagues Keith Engelke, Don Doerr, and Vic Convertino at NASA[10], we found that only an absolutely maximal effort (maximum VO_2) for 15 minutes could prevent the effect of continuous bed rest, though this benefit lasted for no more than 24 hours. It is inconceivable that the average person would be able to maintain a routine of maximal daily exercise for 15 minutes, nor do we know whether this approach done daily would continue to produce these benefits or maybe possibly even have adverse consequences. Bear in mind that health is different from fitness. Health is the absence of disease whereas fitness must be defined by what one is fit to do, presumably with exertion. Problems arise with social expectations about the universal value of exercise. And government guidelines push us in a direction that doesn't necessarily work or solve the sitting problem. The solution is simple, frequent, beneficial daily movement, which is readily available to all anywhere, and is already, to one degree or another, part of our daily lives.

At the beginning of this section, we stated that health is not the same as fitness. Health is how you feel and function. It is usually the absence of disease. Being fit is what you are able to do. Exercise makes you fit for doing something. Often that something involves heavy exertion every once in a while. Moving about all day keeps you healthy. Both are needed. Even after vigorous exercise you need to move. Joints have been stressed and need mobility while they recover or they will stiffen. Moving is the foundation; you cannot live without it. But you can and should build on it with exercise whenever you can. They work in different ways and complement each other. If you only do what is in this book, you may need to add some exercise to gain endurance or strength. But it does not work the other way around. If you only go to the gym for exercise, you may not necessarily be healthy. You still need to build your foundation of good health around all-day moving. It is paying attention to the basics that keeps you healthy and resilient.

All-day activities involve purposeful moving in the course of living. A great many of these movements, like gardening, walking with your friends, walking to the shop, lifting a child, rolling out dough or baking cookies, swinging on a swing, or jumping on a trampoline, are also fun. And they all count toward building and maintaining your health.

The secret is to make it a habit to frequently interrupt those stretches of sitting with smart movements. Habits take about eight weeks to stick and they are free or low cost. Varied and purposeful moving takes away the boredom often associated with exercise. Of course extensive sitting is hard to avoid in our modern world, and it can be made manageable if we develop the habit of interrupting our sitting often enough. But new data shows that as little as one or two hours of uninterrupted sitting can affect how you process your blood sugar, and can increase the risk of cancer, diabetes, and cardiovascular disease, even if you exercise regularly.

Given the popularity of TV and other media, we are encouraged to sit many hours. Jack sits in front of a computer screen all day long. He does not care to exercise because he has back pain but once he understood how that worked, he could go along with the idea of standing up every so often and stretching. It also helped relieve his back pain.

Yes, sitting is now considered an independent risk factor for many chronic diseases as well as for premature death. Even if you smoke like a chimney or are a heavy drinker, or both, it's actually the constant sitting that will do the most damage.

DISPELLING MYTHS

The problem is compounded by perpetuating myths:

- Quickie solutions that a pill or the next medical breakthrough will make us well.

  There is no such thing as a medication or a vitamin that moves for you.

- I can't help it. Long hours of sitting are a necessary part of my workplace because it keeps me electronically connected to my colleagues and customers.

  You can replace electronic communication by physically visiting your office colleagues.

- Outside office hours, extended sitting, whether at home or in cars or trains, is an unavoidable part of modern life.

  Consciously structure breaks that require some form of moving.

- Regular exercise counteracts the impact of uninterrupted sitting.

  Surprisingly, research now shows that this is not the case (as discussed earlier in this chapter).

- Many people don't or cannot keep up a regular exercise program, classes, or even walking.

  Frequent changes in posture can mean just sitting up on a bed with feet dangling over the side or getting help to change posture with a StandUp wheelchair. Staying aligned with gravity and working the upper body throughout the day is quite effective.

- A couple of hours sitting will not harm us.

  Studies show that more than two hours of continuous, uninterrupted sitting, even when combined with regular exercise, are linked with death from breast or colon cancer, increased incidence of diabetes and obesity, heart attacks, and stroke.

- Falls are a sure way to an early death. Balance problems are the cause, not less moving.

  Balance exercises certainly can help strengthen coordination, but how many times a day do you do them? Good balance starts with good gravity-aligned posture, whether standing in line at the post office, grocery shopping, or even sitting.

- Remaining standing for as many hours as you sit is the cure.

  People who need to stand in their jobs suffer from aches, neck and back pain, swollen ankles, and dangerous blood clots in their legs.

It is not the number of hours sat that are the problem, but rather the long hours of sitting without a break that cause poor modern health. Equally, standing for many hours without a break can be just as harmful to one's health as sitting. Ask any person whose job entails being on their feet for many hours, even if they are moving. Think of nurses, those in retail jobs, eating establishments or bars, and painters. Standing is not the opposite of sitting. When you stand, feeling the full vertical force of gravity, your body is fully loaded. When you sit or lie down, you are exposed to reduced vertical gravitational pull; you are "unloading" your body. Your body is designed to require both standing and sitting. Both are essential to good health.

Not only does modern life result in poor health by physical unloading due to too much sitting, but modern technological inventions which flood the market daily are causing mental and emotional overload through incessant stimulation around the clock. The body is unloaded while the brain is overloaded. This formula is sure to spell disaster in the future.

Technological creativity will continue and accelerate. We cannot stop it. We can only learn how to be more discriminating about how we use it, starting from a very early age. Children are particularly vulnerable to this mental bombardment, egged on by constant subtle and not-so-subtle commercial encouragement.

Chapter 3

Causes and Consequences: The Science of Sitting and Standing

Recall from chapters 1 and 2 that bed rest, and especially HDBR, deprives the body of gravity in a similar way to what happens to astronauts in the reduced gravity of space. Similarly, sitting reduces the gravitational pull on the body, though to a lesser extent. We can think of gravity exposure as a continuum, from high exposure when "pulling Gs" in an airplane or riding on a roller coaster, to 1G exposure walking about on Earth, to low exposure when sitting, lying down, or immersed in microgravity during spaceflight. Thus, sitting is a stage along the gravity exposure continuum—a stage in which most of us in modern society spend far too much time. The longer you sit, the faster you deteriorate. Call it aging, illness, disease, or disorder, the effects on your health and how you feel are the same: bad.

How many hours a day do you sit? Who knows? How many people go around counting how many hours they sit each day? You can keep looking at your watch or clock. You can measure how many steps you take with a pedometer. But apart from looking at the clock obsessively, I am not aware of an accurate way to measure how many hours you sit. You only know it is too much when you begin to ache, your back and neck hurt, you feel restless or sluggish, and your brain feels fuzzy and is not functioning at its best.

During my days at medical school in London, the students and faculty took their work/study breaks in a tearoom where there were no chairs. We would stand and chat with one another, much as millions of American office workers used to do around the proverbial watercooler. Our tea breaks were the source of new ideas exchanged and thrashed out, informally meeting scientists from all over the university of all ranks and fields. Today, sadly, the tearoom or watercooler has been replaced by cups of coffee at your desk, leaning back staring at a screen or avatar, slumped in a chair on rollers that obviate even the slightest motion of getting up to reach the printer or a book. Conversation with colleagues is reduced to emails and text messages. A graduate student has to make an appointment to chat with his or her advisor; there is little opportunity to spontaneously share not only their work but their wildest ideas. And when the appointment is made, it involves sitting in the advisor's office. Am I just reminiscing about the good old days? Mostly I am saddened by lost opportunities for human-to-human contact and what that loss might be doing to our intellect and psyche.

THERE'S NO SHORTAGE OF INFORMATION

And yet, it's not that we are unaware of what we are doing to ourselves. It seems that with every new study come new guidelines on what will make us healthier. We are told that we need to eat less and exercise more—but exactly which foods and which kinds of exercise are most beneficial? Every time we look at the news, the advice changes. Perhaps the problem is not a shortage of information, but an overload. Since the field of health is volatile, we are exposed to premature conclusions, oversimplifications, and misunderstandings about what will be effective, and why. Government guidelines can be misguided or confusing since by the time the pertinent advisory group has deliberated and worked it out, the scientific opinion is well dated. Certainly by the time it reaches your personal physician, knowledge has moved on. The same can be true of recommendations from nonprofits and patient-information websites.

Despite knowing that inactivity is harmful, we have allowed ourselves to become victims of a system that wants us to spend our days sitting for work, commuting, communicating through electronics, and so forth. The lack of movement is in turn leading to reduced mobility, pain in the neck or back, stooped posture, muscle and bone weakness, reduced flexibility, and painful joints. Does any of this sound familiar?

Modern medical advances—drugs, surgery, devices—have become a false safety net. The emphasis in medical research is on longevity. We are achieving that. We live longer but not better. How well we will live is not about relegating the care of our health to medicine. It is not about some invading infection that needs to be cured. It requires our personal awareness, to listen to ourselves and what we can do right now, as individuals and as members of the community.

DISTILLING THE DATA

There is, however, one bright spot on the horizon. Thanks to ever more powerful and affordable computers, it has become easier and cheaper to obtain funding for marvelous computer-enabled meta-analyses for epidemiological studies. Anything that uses computers is faster; it speeds up the outpouring of numbers. That's all it does. How you interpret the numbers and the questions you ask of these numbers is where the human intellect comes in. Therefore, a plethora of reports have appeared (and continue to appear) drawing conclusions from correlations of data from unrelated studies between reported hours sat with numerous medical disorders. In the few years since 2010, the number of reports on the sitting problem in scientific journals, the popular press, or TV has exploded. Before discussing the conclusions, it is worth reconsidering what exactly a meta-analysis provides.

Meta-analysis is a statistical process that combines results from different studies to obtain a quantitative estimate of the overall effect of a particular intervention or variable on a defined outcome. For instance, it could be the statistical process for pooling data from many clinical trials to glean a clearer answer that an individual study would not provide. Meta-analysis produces a stronger conclusion than can be provided by any individual study. The larger the number, the stronger is the reliability of the results. However, does it make sense? That would depend on the questions the investigator asks and the reliability of what, when, and how things were measured—not easy for observations made many years previously for a different purpose.

No two studies are identical, so it can be dangerous to ignore any given variable as irrelevant or insignificant. It is more than likely that the analyses are done by statisticians who, excellent as they might be at what they do, mostly have little familiarity or interest in major health variables which would be different and specific to each study but might well impact the outcome. Care must be exercised to avoid the potential for analytical sloppiness through lack of familiarity with the basic physiological issues. Such sloppiness may lead to failure or overstating the strengths and precision of the results.

These comments are not meant to be dismissive of studies using meta-analysis as long as they are not used as the ultimate proof. Meta-analysis, in fact, may be used as a general guide to perhaps set a hypothesis that would be followed by more carefully controlled research to confirm preliminary findings. Alternatively, it may be used following preliminary research that would underscore the importance of relevant variables in a larger pool of subjects.

Most of the current findings on the overall public ills of sitting are based on meta-analyses. Overall, few well-controlled studies of cause and effect have been carried out to date. These have dealt mostly with diabetes markers and some cardiovascular measures that change fairly rapidly in response to sitting, chronic habitual sitting in front of a computer or TV, or occupational sitting conditions, such as in the office environment. Here the knowledge gleaned from using the tightly controlled bed-rest analog of spaceflight comes in useful for studies of lengthier periods of lying down. After all, in the real world, most of us are concerned about daily sedentary behaviors of many hours per day, over months or years. In this respect, meta-analyses may be more indicative of long-term public health issues.

How sedentary behavior is measured may vary from study to study, with most being self-reported. Relying on memory or general perception of how many hours one sits can be inaccurate. I can attest to this as I sit at the computer to write on a daily basis, and I find when I get on a roll that I am sitting much longer at a stretch, whether my timing buzzer goes off or not. I'll say to myself, "Surely half an hour more is not going to make too much difference! After all, I was the one who created this national moving movement, so I must get some 'free' extra time!" Or, I might argue that using my fingers to type and my brain to think and convert ideas to written words may be just as good in increasing my brain blood flow as standing up every thirty minutes. I do not believe it, but until proven otherwise maybe I can get away with cheating my body. I imagine most of us make similar rationalizations from time to time in our lives.

Evaluating the information of meta-analysis studies therefore depends on how sedentary behavior is defined by each one of us, how it is recalled—sometimes after years—and how it is measured. Brigid Lynch and Neville Owen from the IDI Baker Institute in Melbourne, Australia[11], emphasized the importance of conducting research using device-based measurement rather than self-reporting, as was used in many early studies. I will have more to say about the Australian research later in the chapter.

There have also been some excellent studies that accurately set the scene of today's sitting human, detailing health consequences, what goes wrong, and how it can be fixed. I shall distill the data for you, providing you with what you need to know to make good choices about your daily life, even if you have a lifestyle today that seems to discourage movement. The world has changed around you, in the way you live, work, and play. We need to catch up. First, become aware of the ways in which a sedentary lifestyle can be harmful; next, readjust your life habits to sail through to health and happiness.

HEALTH PROBLEMS RELATED TO SITTING

Most of us spend as much as 55 percent or more of our waking hours each day sitting. We sit at the table during meals, we sit while driving our cars, we sit working at a desk at the office or at school, and we finish off the day sitting on the couch watching TV in the evening. According to the American Heart Association[12], sedentary jobs have risen 83 percent since 1950; today less than 20 percent of all jobs in the United States involve any serious degree of physical activity.

A growing number of studies show that the more we sit, the greater our chances of dying of heart disease, stroke, cancer, or diabetes. We tend to get back and joint pain. We are likely to be overweight or obese. Sitting also saps our energy, making us more tired than ever. In a commentary titled "Regular Physical Activity: Forgotten Benefits," published in 2015 online in the *American Journal of Medicine*, Drs. Steven Lewis and Charles Hennekins of Florida Atlantic University stress that lack of physical activity in Americans poses important clinical, public health, and fiscal challenges for the nation. They calculate that the cost of habitual inactivity and the resultant poor health ". . . accounts for 22% of coronary heart disease, 22% of colon cancer, 18% of osteoporotic fractures, 12% of diabetes and hyper-tension, and 5% of breast cancer . . . . inactivity accounts for about 2.4% of U.S. healthcare expenditures or approximately \$24 billion a year."[13] Not a pretty picture.

As the data continue to come in, certain patterns emerge. Dorothy Dunlap at Northwestern University[5] discovered that in 60-year-olds that even a small increase in sitting time could be debilitating. For instance, sitting for 13 hours a day was 50 percent more likely to be disabling than sitting for 12 hours. In other words, after many hours of sitting, a smaller increase in sitting time produces a disproportionately bigger risk. Another study found that high amounts of sitting time (16 hours per day or more) were associated with cardiovascular events (both fatal and nonfatal) in post-menopausal women.[14] A Finnish meta-analysis study of 22,518 persons' data found an approximately 40% greater risk of coronary heart disease in employees working over five hours per day.[15] In general, it appears that anything longer than three hours per day can increase health risks, and certainly over eight hours per day is in the danger zone.

My research with bed-rest volunteers suggests that interrupting lying down at regular intervals will prevent the adverse effects.[9] Similarly, we can predict that standing up at regular intervals will prevent the adverse effects of continuous sitting. If indeed sitting is merely a stage along the gravity exposure continuum, then the effects of too much sitting should be similar, though quantitatively different, to what is seen in astronauts in space, volunteers in bed rest, and ordinary humans on Earth as we age (check back with Table 1 in Chapter 1). However, the data I will discuss in this section are from actual sitting studies in humans.

Mortality: does sitting really kill?

The case is made concerning hours spent sitting and its relationship to mortality. The World Health Organization (WHO) estimates 3.3 to 5 million people die annually due to physical inactivity, making it the fourth leading cause of mortality.

Longevity studies, such as the Baltimore Longitudinal Aging Study and the National Health and Nutrition Examination Survey (NHANES), were both initiated in the late 1950s to follow changes in aging and nutritional practices respectively in normal humans. In the 1970s, questions on exercise and fitness levels began to be noted. Attention to hours spent sitting was not a priority in those early days—I doubt they are now—and relied heavily on recall of habits. Surviving participants may be asked to recall such habits. Nevertheless, meta-analysis techniques are very useful in such longitudinal studies that may be better controlled in general than the occasional survey. For example, an analysis of 18 studies[16] found that people who sat for the longest periods of time were twice as likely to have diabetes or heart disease, compared to those who sat the least. The risk for greatest sitting time compared with the lowest was 112 percent greater for diabetes, 147 percent greater for cardiovascular events, 90 percent more for mortality from cardiovascular disease, and 49 percent more for all-cause mortality. Such a 50 percent increase in mortality by all causes is serious by any measure.

Some seminal studies have set the scene with respect to the relationship of sitting time and mortality or disease prediction. Earlier studies on the effects of sitting focused on the number of hours of TV watching, since it was easier for people to recall how many hours they might have watched TV than how many hours they spent sitting. In 2009, Peter Katzmarzyk at the Pennington Research Center in Baton Rouge, LA, reported the dangers of excessive hours of TV-watching on cardiovascular disease, cancer, and overall mortality.[17]

Charles Matthews at the National Cancer Institute in Rockville, MD, and his collaborators in 2012 published data from 240,819 adults aged 50 to 71 who participated in the NIH-AARP Diet and Health Study.[18] They started out symptom-free and were assessed 8.5 years later. Sedentary behaviors, including watching TV for more than seven hours per day, as compared with less than one hour per day, were most strongly associated with mortality from all causes, as well as cardiovascular mortality specifically. Interestingly, moderate to vigorous physical activity did not help much. As I have pointed out previously and will explain further in this chapter, we cannot counteract the damage that results from sitting all day by exercising for an hour.

Dr. David Dunstan (from the Baker IDI Heart and Diabetes Institute, Melbourne, Australia), the senior leader of a multi-institutional, multinational team, led a study of 200,000 Australians aged 45 and older who were observed over three years and monitored with activity devices.[19] During this period around 5,000 of them died. About 7 percent of the deaths were associated with prolonged sitting. Those who sat longer than 11 hours per day had a 40 percent greater risk of dying compared to people who sat for less than four hours. Those who sat for eight or more hours per day had a 15 percent increased risk of dying. Other risk factors such as age and smoking did not influence these results.

CANCER

There have been several meta-analysis studies reporting increased occurrence as well as risk of various forms of cancer as a function of sedentary behavior. These data are consistent, though they remain limited because of the many varieties of cancer as well as insufficient attention to other factors that may co-exist in their sitting populations. These might include obesity, diabetes, and cardiovascular disease. In 2007, Brigid Lynch, while still at the Alberta Health Services in Calgary, Canada, comprehensively reviewed the existing literature on sedentary behavior and cancer.[20] She drew significant associations with colorectal and digestive tract, endometrial, ovarian, breast, and prostate cancers. In a review of 70,000 cancer cases, Daniela Schmid and Michael Leitzman of the University of Regensburg in Germany found that sitting was associated with a 24 percent increased risk of colon cancer, a 32 percent increased risk of endometrial cancer, and a 21 percent increased risk of lung cancer. They note that, contrary to the general public's expectations, "you cannot exercise away the habit's harmful effects . . . . Even participants who achieved the daily recommended levels of physical activity were at the same risk as those who spent their day sitting."[21] Peter Katzmaryk's research with colleagues at the Pennington in Baton Rouge, Louisiana, in 2009, further showed that there was a dose-response relationship between sitting time and mortality from all causes, including cancer.[17] The World Health Organization (WHO) report in 2014 predicted a 70 percent increase in cancers over the next twenty years from infection or lifestyle. I find it fascinating that lifestyle is up there with infection with respect to cancer; at least lifestyle is something over which we can take control.

REPRODUCTIVE DISORDERS

Sitting time has been found to increase the risk of disturbed reproductive function and health. Erectile dysfunction and increased odds of benign hyperplasia of the prostate have been reported with a higher risk when sitting exceeded seven hours per day, whereas reducing sedentary time could have a protective effect. Studies with larger numbers of participants are needed to validate these important observations. Nevertheless, would the potential benefits of a better sex life, in addition to better health in general, not be worth the effort of curtailing sitting time?

CARDIOVASCULAR DISORDERS

Exercise has been the treatment of choice for cardiovascular health and function. Therefore, it was assumed that sitting, by removing activity, had adverse effects on cardiovascular health. More recent studies that have measured the contribution of sitting to cardiovascular health have added a new dimension.

Jacquelin Kulinski at the Medical College of Wisconsin used CT heart scans to monitor calcium ion plaque as it accumulated over time, causing the arteries to narrow.[22] Participants sat for an average of two to 12 hours with an average of five hours. Monitored CT heart scan activity meter records (accelerometers) found that each additional hour of sedentary time per day was associated with a 14 percent increase in coronary artery calcification, whether or not the patient exercised or practiced other traditional heart disease preventive treatment.

As in astronauts and bed–rest volunteers, the endothelial lining of veins is affected by too much sitting. Saurabh Thosar and colleagues at the University of Indiana reported that as little as one to three hours of sitting decreases the shear forces in the superficial femoral vein and decreases the endothelial lining of the vein, a marker of atherosclerotic cardiovascular disease.[23] Within just one hour of sitting, there was a large (about 50 percent) drop in artery dilation and reduction in the shear rate of blood flow in the blood vessel. Interestingly, this effect was restored or prevented by a single hourly bout of mild walking at the pace of just two miles per hour.

Risk of heart failure is another cardiovascular consequence of too much sitting. An extensive sedentary time analysis over almost eight years was carried out in a very large group of patients—82,695 men aged over the age of 45—by the Kaiser Permanente hospital system in California.[24] The results showed a direct relationship between the incidents of heart failure and the hours of sitting. In patients who sat for five, three, or two hours per day, roughly eight, five, and 3.8 incidents, respectively, of heart failure per 1,000 persons were observed. The more hours of sitting, the higher was the risk of heart failure.

Sedentary habits and overall tendency to be inactive have also been implicated in the incidence of a first ever stroke. Factors such as a diet which contribute to higher triglycerides may be expected to act synergistically with sitting habits to increase the risk of cardiovascular disease.

It is clear that exercise is important in reducing your overall cardiovascular risk as well as improving your fitness level. But study after study suggest that reducing how many hours you sit continuously every day may represent a more relevant factor than exercise.

METABOLISM

Metabolism is a pattern of chemical reactions in the body's cells that convert fuel from the food we eat (i.e., calories) into the energy we need to move our muscles. Muscle is the chemical factory of the body. It generates the body's energy needs. If your muscle does not move, does not contract, you will have less energy. Sitting is a great example of where by default your muscle is not contracting because it is not stimulated by movement. Under those conditions it begins to atrophy. The signal your muscle receives is that it is no longer needed. The result is that protein synthesis stops, followed by greater protein breakdown and muscle loss. Fat stores increase and infiltrate the muscle.

When you are sitting, energy requirements are reduced to a basal metabolic rate that is just enough to take care of any small residual movement and to maintain body temperature. The resistance of muscle to insulin appears almost immediately when you sit or lie down in bed during the day. A glucose or carbohydrate meal is used to test for insulin resistance. Insulin resistance is measurable within 30 minutes after a glucose meal in persons who have been sitting. Insulin resistance, glucose intolerance, and triglycerides all increased, whereas fasting insulin, glucose, and lipid levels (HDL and LDL) were unaltered over the seven day sitting period studied.[25]

In 2012, the Centers for Disease Control (CDC) estimated that there were 29 million Type-2 diabetics in the U.S. and that number was rising rapidly. Type-2 diabetes is characterized by insulin resistance in the presence of reduced or inadequate insulin; that is, the body cannot maintain the blood glucose within normal limits. Obese individuals may also have insulin resistance, with probably more insulin produced by the pancreas in an effort to overcome the resistance and maintain the blood sugar near normal. Known as a pre-diabetic state, high insulin levels cause greater accumulation of fat and massive inflammation. As the pancreas can no longer maintain the needed high insulin levels, those levels eventually drop, resulting in high circulating glucose and Type-2 diabetes. Not all obese individuals have insulin resistance and therefore do not become diabetic. Results of the EPIC study (European Prospective Investigation into Cancer and Nutrition) showed that, out of the 9.2 million deaths in Europe over about 12 years, twice as many deaths were due to inactivity (676,000) as those from obesity (337,000).[26]

Sitting changes metabolism. Not only does insulin resistance not allow glucose to enter muscle to be used as fuel, but triglycerides are increased as there is a decreased ability to use fats for energy, even in healthy young men. Lionel Bey and Marc Hamilton, when at the University of Missouri, found that inactivity in mice decreased the enzyme lipoprotein lipase in the blood, allowing fat to accumulate.[27] Subsequently, David Dustan and his colleagues showed the same thing in sitting men.[19] This reaction is not gradual; triglycerides are increased within 30 minutes of sitting. In contrast, standing up and moving about does the opposite: It promptly increases the circulating levels of lipoprotein lipase and relieves insulin resistance.[28] Audrey Bergouignan and her colleagues found that being inactive by lying in bed also results in decreased high density lipoproteins (HDL; "good" cholesterol) and increased low density lipoproteins (LDL; "bad" cholesterol).[29]

If you were concerned that too much sitting was making you gain weight, you are not wrong. Unused fat has to go somewhere. But it does not just collect under your skin. If you do not move, fat finds its way into bone and, even worse, into the kidneys and the liver, where it can affect their function. It is probable that fat also accumulates in heart muscle, though the data are too preliminary on that score to draw a definite connection.

The more hours you sit, the more muscle strength, energy, quantity and quality of muscle mass, and metabolic function all go downhill. Eventually, persistent long hours of sitting lead to progressively more muscle loss with age. In turn, muscle loss means losing mobility, balance, coordination, and independence. You become frail. You have a greater chance of falling and being injured.

THE BRAIN AND COGNITIVE FUNCTION

I have just listed many ways in which excessive sitting is detrimental to your physical health, but let's not leave out what it does to your mental health. Just like the rest of your body, your brain depends on blood supply from adequate blood flow to provide it with oxygen, glucose, and other nutrients. When you are sitting, blood flow to the brain is reduced. The longer you sit, the more likely it is that your blood will pool to your feet rather than get to your head where it is needed for your brain to function.

Depending on how long you sit, the impact of such reduced blood flow to your brain becomes progressively worse. Such deprivation not only affects your brain functions—thinking, memory, sleeping, and even breathing—but cumulative deprivation over a long period of time can have disastrous effects on cognitive function. From age 20 on, when development peaks, we sit more and move less. It stands to reason that we progressively deprive our brain of essentials for normal function. It is therefore not too surprising that sitting is now linked with all aspects of brain function, including how you think and feel.

An Australian study, published in *Epidemiology & Prevention*, set out to determine if prolonged sitting and lack of exercise have an effect on depression.[30] Researchers analyzed the habits of nearly 9,000 women, ages 50 to 55, over several years. Women who sat for more than seven hours per day were found to have a 47 percent higher risk of depression than women who sat for four hours or less per day. It is ironic that one of the consequences of depression is increased sitting. It is a vicious cycle. Other researchers have come to similar conclusions about the mental effects of sitting. British researchers found that spending leisure time on the computer and watching TV were associated with reduced feelings of well-being. A study of more than 3,000 government workers in Australia found those who spent more than six hours seated per workday were more likely to score higher in psychological distress than those sitting fewer than three hours, regardless of how active they were outside of work.[16]

Why does sitting have such a negative impact on your mental health? *Psychology Today* concludes it may have to do with what people tend to do while in their chairs.

> Some of the psychological effects of sitting may be rooted in what they do. They may stare at an electronic screen, rather than connecting emotionally with others. They may watch mindless TV shows, rather than engaging intellectually with the world. Or they may multitask ceaselessly—flitting between work emails, personal texts, social media, and the Internet—rather than honing their attention.[31]

Spending excess time at your computer may lead to insomnia and depression. A British study involving 25,000 people found that those working long hours in front of computers complained of feeling depressed, anxious, and reluctant to get up for work in the mornings. They found that working just five hours per day in front of a computer screen was enough to produce depression and insomnia.[32] Sedentary habits can take their toll on executive analysis and decision-making. In fact, executive dysfunction is directly related to hours spent sitting rather than, say, smoking or drinking.

Sitting also affects the structure of the brain. The most common observations of the physical consequences of sedentary behavior on the brain relate both to anatomy as well as to functions such as balance and coordination. Dr. Utho Kujala, Professor of Sports and Exercise Medicine at the University of Jyvaskyla, Finland, and his team studied ten pairs of Finnish twins, in which one of each set of twins was sedentary and the other more active. He found that the sedentary twins had less gray matter in the part of their brains that is mostly involved in motor control and coordination than their more active twin. They also had lower endurance capacities and higher proportion of body fat and signs of insulin resistance, in spite of similar diets, suggesting that food choices were unlikely to contribute to these health differences.[33]

White matter is brain tissue containing nerve fibers responsible for brain communication. As we age, nerve fiber activity decreases and disrupts brain function. The structural integrity of white matter not only relies on physical activity but is also affected by the amount of time spent sitting.

A team of investigators at the China Astronaut Research and Training Centre in Beijing used MRI to measure changes in brain gray matter in fourteen volunteers lying continuously in bed for thirty days. Gray matter volume decreased in, among other sites, the bilateral frontal cortex lobes, temporal lobes, and the right hippocampus, accompanied by some fractional changes in white matter tracts. Such regions in gray matter are closely associated with performance, locomotion, learning, memory, and coordination. Regional white matter changes would be expected to be related to brain function decline and adaptation. Movement and coordination changes would have been expected, but the changes in the other regions were recorded for the first time, providing neuro-anatomical evidence of brain dysfunction and a deeper insight into brain mechanisms and how they are affected by prolonged sitting. What was surprising was how rapidly these changes appeared.[34]

BALANCE AND COORDINATION

The inner ear, located near the center of the brain, controls balance and coordination. It gives us our sense of direction and speed. You may have noticed that spending a few days in bed with the flu is enough to make you unsteady when you get out of bed again, and it's not just your imagination. Astronauts returning from space where there is no up or down because of the reduced gravity environment show problems with maintaining their balance and coordinating their movements; the same thing happens with healthy bed-rest volunteers getting out of bed after as little as seven days. Their stance and gait show obvious problems, with feet wider apart than usual and shorter steps taken. They walk more like a one-year-old toddler or a shuffling old person. They may have trouble negotiating corners—walking briskly down a hallway and unexpectedly bumping into the wall when it comes time to make a turn into a doorway or another hallway. During testing for balance after only seven days on the shuttle in 1993, pilot Rick Searfoss suddenly fell straight forward, only to be grabbed by bystanders who stopped him from hitting the ground. He had made no gesture to protect his fall, nor, as he told us, did he experience any sensation that he was falling! It was an eye-opener. How could such a radical change happen in just seven days, such a short period of time? We did not know if, when, and whether he would recover. Fortunately, he did, as did others after him, once they resumed their normal lives, but we developed a harness to protect future astronauts from falling during this test.

DEMENTIA

Higher levels of exercise have been claimed to improve signs of early dementia, but the results remain inconclusive. The fact that some studies rely on what patients say or think they do, and others on what they actually do, leads to a great deal of inconsistency. In a study of adults age 60 to 80, Agnieszka Burzynska and colleagues at the University of Illinois used accelerometers to monitor physical activity continuously for seven days. They also mapped lesions in the white matter with brain imaging. Such lesions are not uncommon in older individuals, such as those in this study. The results showed fewer lesions in those who engaged in low-level physical exercise. However, those who did only light physical activity had even greater structural benefit in their white matter of the temporal lobes, which play a prominent role in memory, language, sight, and hearing.

Most interesting was that those who sat the most hours, even if they exercised at the end of the day for half an hour, suffered detrimental effects on the white matter of their hippocampus, the brain region most important to memory and learning. Exercise had not prevented the effects on the brain that come from prolonged sitting.[35]

BACK PAIN

We seem to live in an era of back pain. Sitting all day or even moving from one seat to another does not help the pain. It would be inaccurate to pretend that pain directly causes death. However, medications—so-called painkillers—do, either through overuse, the need for ever increasing doses, or, in the case of opioids, through the addiction they cause. An incredible selection of synthetic opiate analgesics as well as steroid injections and non-steroidal anti-inflammatories are now used for pain of all types, but predominantly for back pain. When pharmaceuticals do not resolve the pain, support devices and back surgery provide temporary relief since in most cases the root cause—sitting—persists.

WHO ARE MOST VULNERABLE?

It seems that the most vulnerable to the ill effects of too much sitting are children, the elderly, patients in intensive care units (ICUs), older post-orthopedic surgery patients (such as after hip or knee surgery), and in those where mobility is inherently reduced. Sitting seems particularly impactful in conditions where the rate of change in basic metabolism is at its highest—at least the effects of sitting become more evident in those conditions.

CHILDREN

Anyone who spends even short periods of time with young children knows that they have an amazing amount of energy and are by nature constantly moving. During the first five to ten years of development, their basic metabolism is changing at a very high rate, for their young bodies need energy not just for movement and internal functions like blood circulation and nervous system reactions, but also for the growth of muscles, bones, nerve fibers, and so forth. Yet as adults we often find children's constant moving about to be an annoyance. It can be tempting to park children in front of the TV or video game console and instruct them to sit still for however long is convenient for the adult.

For many years, the American Academy of Pediatrics has recommended no more than two hours a day of entertainment screen time (television, computer, etc.) for children aged two and older, noting that "It is important for kids to spend time on outdoor play, reading, hobbies, and using their imaginations in free play." And for infants and toddlers under age two, the academy recommends no screen time at all because "A child's brain develops rapidly during these first years, and young children learn best by interacting with people, not screens." Sadly, the average amount of time children actually spend in front of the screen is seven hours per day.

Increasingly, research is confirming that sitting in front of a computer is bad for children in a variety of ways. Mark de Boer from the University of Virginia presented at the Pediatric Society in San Diego the results of a survey of 11,113 kindergartners and first-graders during the 2011–2012 school year who watched even as little as one hour of TV per day. They were more likely to be overweight or obese, then and later, than children who watched less TV.[36] Valerie Strauss notes:

> We quickly learned after further testing that most of the children in the classroom had poor core strength and balance. In fact, we tested a few other classrooms and found that when compared to children from the early 1980s, only one out of twelve children had normal strength and balance. Only one! Oh my goodness, I thought to myself. These children need to move![37]

With the availability of "sitting still" screen entertainments, it is no wonder that American children get too little opportunity to move about. In fact, the *2014 United States Report Card on Physical Activity for Children and Youth* gave them a D– overall, and a D for sedentary behaviors. It found that children were spending more than seven hours per day at sedentary activities.[38] A 2013 poll by the Harvard School of Public Health found that "almost seven in 10 parents say their child's school does not provide daily physical education, even though experts recommend 150 to 225 minutes per school week."[39]

In spite of sport or exercise, screen viewing on weekends was associated with loss of bone density in boys, though less so in girls. It turns out that the boys spent more time in front of screens than girls, averaging five hours per day on weekends and about four hours per day during the week. The equivalent time for girls was four hours during weekends and just over three hours during the week. It also turns out that this bone loss in boys was in spite of four hours per week of hard training for competitive sports. In other research, children who spent four hours or more computer-gaming reported feeling less well than their friends who spent less time in this activity. Children spending more time in front of computer screens also had more emotional problems, anxiety, depression, and behavioral difficulties.

If you observe the entrance to a local school in the morning when children are arriving, you are likely to see a long line of cars waiting to get into the drop-off area. While some children travel to school by bus, those who are not served by school bus routes are routinely driven in private cars. Letting a child walk to school has become almost unheard of in many communities, even for children who live within a block or two of the school.

Once in the school environment, children are often encouraged or even required to sit still as part of learning to pay attention. The traditional 40-minute or one-hour block of instruction time may just require too much sitting. Children who spend hours sitting are bored, restless, depressed, and now show up with diabetes, heart conditions, stroke, obesity, and other signs of poor health.[40] These conditions used to be seen first in people over 50, not in children.

It has already been well established that insufficient physical activity is significantly contributing to our national epidemic of childhood obesity. [37] A mammoth NIH study in 2015 tested children who were between ages seven and 11.[41] (Nearly 17 percent of children and teens were obese, according to the Endocrine Society's *Facts and Figures* report. If your child spends a lot of time in front of an electronic screen, his or her mental health may also be at risk. In one UK study, excessive screen time produced negative effects on children's self-worth, self-esteem, and level of self-reported happiness. In contrast, St. Finian's, an elementary school in Sterling, Scotland, instituted a "daily walk or run a mile between classes" to improve the students' health and focus their minds. After three years the program claims none of their students were overweight.

Charles Hillman of the University of Illinois comments:

> Physically active children also have increased concentration and enhanced attention spans when compared to their less active peers. The authors find that fitness is related to the ability to inhibit attention to competing stimuli during a task, an ability that can help children stay focused and persevere to complete an assignment. The findings on attention encompass children with special needs as well as typically developing children . . . . [Physical activity can be effective] as a non-pharmaceutical intervention for children with attention-deficit-hyperactivity disorder and children with autism spectrum disorders, with positive results.[42]

However, the emphasis to be explored should be on sedentary hours rather than the physical activity.

It is also important to recognize that the spontaneous activity of a child is nothing like the structured physical activity provided in a school curriculum. G.D. Myers, Director of Research at The Human Performance Laboratory for the Division of Sports Medicine at Cincinnati Children's Hospital Medical Center, and his team point out that current recommendations for physical activity overlook the critical importance of motor skills acquired naturally early in life. Instead, they focus on quantifying how much physical activity children should engage in (e.g. sixty minutes of daily moderate to vigorous physical activity, aerobic fitness, muscular strength, muscular endurance, flexibility, and body composition).[43]

This is not the way nature works. Focusing on exercise quantity ignores qualitative aspects, such as developing skills in a playful social context for the purpose of enjoyment. Preadolescence is a critical time for skill learning and developing and reinforcing motor skills. Boys and girls who do not exercise motor skills during childhood may never reach their genetic potential for motor skill control, which is the foundation for sustained physical fitness later in life.

To overcome this, a good place to start is to observe spontaneous activities that children indulge in. Spontaneous activity deals mostly with gravity-using play like tumbling, hopping, directional changes, and balance and coordination activities such as juggling, turning cartwheels, riding a bicycle, roller-blading, jumping on a trampoline, skating, or skiing. These are not likely to be taught in a physical education class. It is time to challenge and reconsider the current dogma of physical activity recommendations for youth.

However, there is also good news. Interrupting a long period of sitting with three-minute breaks every 30 minutes to walk on a treadmill can have immediate effects on a child's metabolism, due to its ability to control blood sugar and insulin levels better than uninterrupted sitting. The key factor here is that it was interrupting sitting frequently that was most effective. It is my belief that less than three minutes would have been equally effective. Learning from children, when Eriek Peper at San Francisco State University is lecturing in the classroom, he has his college students stand up every 30 minutes and wave their arms above their heads before sitting down again when he resumes his lecture. He claims that this short break helps to keep their cognitive skills sharp.[44]

As I was growing up, we would be expected to stand up when a teacher entered the room and when she left. In France, then-president Nicolas Sarkozy (2007–2012) proposed reinstating this practice in French schools. Do your sums and you can see how this elaborate NIH study (see above) did the science behind such practices. No treadmill required.

Workplace sitting

Once we finish school, we move on to become members of the workforce, where most of us are expected to sit for even longer stretches of time without a break. Yet, growing evidence points to the fact that people who sit all day—even if they're active outside of work—are at increased risk for serious health conditions, such as multiple chronic diseases and poorer cognitive and mental function. As mentioned earlier in this chapter, sedentary jobs have risen 83 percent since 1950 and currently account for 43 percent of all jobs in the United States. The American Heart Association also points out that the traditional 40-hour work week is no longer the norm, as those who have a full-time job in the U.S. work about 47 hours per week.[12] There goes the idea of Saturdays spent taking a hike or playing sports! The World Health Organization (WHO) estimates 3.3 to 5 million people die annually due to physical inactivity, making it the fourth leading cause of mortality.

Sitting has been called the ticking timebomb of office desk jobs. The impact of excessive sitting in front of a computer screen in the office has no less important implications to individual health, as well as personal and organizational productivity (and related costs), than it does in the schoolroom. Organizations have tackled this issue by providing onsite gyms or offsite gym memberships for employees, encouraging them to take advantage of these facilities and opportunities. Lucas Carr's research at the University of Iowa has found that, indeed, the best way to get people moving at work is to change the environment in such a way that makes being active easier—a strategy his latest study shows can pay off for both employees and their employers. "But," says Carr "a lot of companies have gone the route of building expensive fitness facilities that typically get used only by the most healthy employees. The people who need to improve their health the most are less likely to use worksite fitness facilities."[45]

Some companies even encourage the wearing of pedometers or other such devices to monitor progress and health, although some have expressed concerns that this invades personal privacy. Tim Cooke, CEO of Apple, was criticized for emphasizing such health benefits on the launch of the Apple watch. Nevertheless, business analysts argue that workplace wellness programs should be explored to cut chronic illness costs.

Based on the present data, encouraging individuals, whether at work or home, to move as much as possible, especially in maintaining good posture and frequently changing their posture, should result in significant health benefits. One way to do this, especially for employees who are reluctant to exercise, is to provide the employee with an option to be active right at their desk. And let's not forget the hours before and after that it takes to get to and from work—sitting on a long commute while driving a car or while riding on a train or bus seat—this all has to be factored in by any employer. While working at home arrangements could allow more freedom to get up from the desk at regular intervals, they do not automatically mean that a worker would sit any less.

What about people who cannot stand up? In addition to losing their independence, are persons with spinal cord injury (SCI) doomed to continuing poor health from the same consequences of a sedentary life that able-bodied people suffer? It used to be that SCIs were condemned to spending a lifetime in bed, since they would faint when they sat up. It was recognized by the mid-twentieth century that this did not have to be so. This fainting tendency could be overcome by repeated changes in posture from lying down to sitting up—just as able-bodied bed-ridden patients recover after surgery, for instance. Post-operative recovery, rehabilitation, and better health resulted in reduced medical costs as well. Now, stand-up wheelchairs enable people with spinal cord injuries and recovering patients to stand up, providing support as well as some mobility and bringing the healing benefits that standing up provides to able-bodied persons.

Reduction in health insurance premiums would be yet another mechanism for motivation, just as it was effectively used to encourage employees in the national initiative to stop smoking. When it comes to sitting, it is not quite as simple to implement because accurate measuring devices of hours sitting or consensus on the most effective interventions needed are not quite established yet.

Reducing the total number of hours spent sitting is not practical in an environment that depends heavily on screen time. Pedometers do not provide the relevant information, nor is exercising regularly in a gym the agreed solution. As good as structured exercise once a day might be for strength and endurance, it does not counteract the consequences of too much sitting the rest of the time. The correct device must measure accurately the variable that directly relates to the problem. As far as we currently know, that would need to be a non-invasive continuous monitor of posture. And/or we could restructure the design of the workplace environment to provide opportunities to change posture and discourage prolonged sitting. This is not as far-fetched as it sounds at first, and it is beginning to be put to the test in a few places (e.g. Google). The Commonwealth Bank of Sydney, Australia, has removed desks and phone landlines. You have to go up a floor to get to a conference room. Employees sit no more than fifteen minutes at any time and feel energized. This approach builds greater cultural cohesion and saves on operating costs.

Changing the practices or design of an organization depends on the quality of its leadership and the examples the leaders set. At one of my talks at a nursing home in Steamboat Springs, Colorado, I met a very elegant lady named Ann Martin who told me she had worked as a steno-typist for the CEO of Met Life in New York City until the 1970s. Now 102, she told of company rules that required all employees to stand up at 11 a.m. and 3 p.m., move to the open window (they had windows in the Met Life building in New York City at that time that could be opened and closed by hand!), stretch up, wave arms around, breathe deeply, and return to one's desk. Though this may not sound like much, in her case she also got up and moved from and back to her desk several times a day as the boss called on her. Together with getting up to have a drink of water at the water fountain and using the restroom, she naturally interrupted her sitting many times each day without a second thought.

A young man at one of my talks objected to my comments, saying he would be fired if he stood up every thirty minutes. "Do you go to the water fountain for water?" "We do not have water fountains; but I have a bottle of water on my desk." "Great. Move your bottle at arm's length away to the next desk or put it on a high shelf so that you have to stand up when you need to drink." It comes down to becoming aware of your environment and restructuring your routine to include opportunities to stand, whether it is walking up to a colleague for information instead of messaging or just to say hello. A friend who is a business coach once told me that if you stand up and smile when making a phone call, your voice will sound better. Whether this leads to business success or not, it provides another good reason to take a "stand-up break" at work.

For nine years at my Washington, D.C., NASA job, I held "ten-minute all-hands stand-up" meetings every morning. After initial complaining and moaning, this custom became popular and copied. Everyone was included and no one gave long-winded comments. Besides, as it turned out, it was good for everyone's health.

Sara Rosenkrantz of Kansas State University agrees with me in that the critical factor to maintaining good health in the workplace depends on how many times and how often sitting is interrupted—in other words, how often there is a posture change.[46] The measures of insulin sensitivity, lipoprotein lipase, and triglycerides that were used in her studies are all useful, reliable markers of when and how well or poorly the intervention is working in preventing the adverse effects of sitting. This information is far more useful than merely recording total time spent sitting. But there is as yet no continuous non-invasive methodology available for monitoring such changes.

Fatigue score was greater when sitting all day than with standing up breaks. Continuous sitting is very hard on the back and back pain is a serious consequence of sitting, resulting in absenteeism in the workplace. Intermittent sit-stand protocols, thirty minutes of on-off standing and sitting, prevented these effects of continuing sitting in obese and over-weight individuals who were sitting for a total of eight hours in an office setting. Also measured were relieved muscle and joint pain, focus, and productivity. Emily Mailey, co-author and director of the Physical Activity Lab, also agrees: "When it comes to sitting time, frequent interruptions is what's really important. We want to break up those long, prolonged bouts of sitting and get people up and moving more throughout the day."[46] Tailoring these intervals to each individual's health/sitting profile would be the ultimate solution. My own preference would be a personal Interrupt Sitting Score (ISS) punch card-like app where the number of interruptions would be cumulatively recorded. The app would also tell you how long you sat before moving again, with green and red lights flashing and buzzing or playing some peppy music to get you going. We jump when the phone rings or when we receive a new email—why not literally jump up?

"The assumption has been that if you're fit and physically active, that will protect you, even if you spend a huge amount of time sitting each day," said Rebecca Seguin, assistant professor of nutritional sciences in Cornell's College of Human Ecology. "In fact, in doing so you are far less protected from the negative health effects of being sedentary than you realize."[47]

A humorous article in *The Onion* titled "Health Experts Recommend Standing Up At Desk, Leaving Office, Never Coming Back," quoted this tongue-in-cheek advice from the Mayo Clinic:

> "Many Americans spend a minimum of eight hours per day sitting in an office, but we observed significant physical and mental health benefits in subjects after just one instance of standing up, walking out the door, and never coming back to their place of work again," said researcher Claudine

Sparks, who explained that those who implemented the practice in their lives reported an improvement in mood and reduced stress that lasted for the remainder of the day, and which appeared to persist even into subsequent weeks. "We encourage Americans to experiment with stretching their legs by strolling across their office and leaving all their responsibilities behind forever just one time to see how much better they feel. People tend to become more productive, motivated, and happy almost immediately. We found that you can also really get the blood flowing by pairing this activity with hurling your staff ID across the parking lot." Sparks added that Americans could maximize positive effects by using their lunch break to walk until nothing looks familiar anymore and your old life is a distant memory.[48]

Perhaps that's a bit extreme, but anything that gets people up and moving is a good thing. People do not move enough whether at work or at home. "Our entire culture has become more sedentary. Physical activity has been engineered out of people's lives," says Dr. Russell Leupker, Mayo Professor of Public Health and expert in Community and Global Health. "We put employees in smaller and smaller cubicles in front of a computer screen and they sit there all day."[49]

It is no longer a question of merely keeping employees happy and healthy. Taking control of the office sitting problem also has important practical, social, and financial implications for workplaces.

OLDER ADULTS

As life expectancy in the United States continues to rise, maintaining physical independence among older adults has also emerged as a major clinical and public health priority. A critical factor in an older person's ability to function independently depends on how well they move without assistance. Older adults who lose mobility are less likely to remain living alone, in their home and in their community. This is a crucial factor in maintaining their sense of identity, self-confidence, and independence. The result is a steeper downhill slope in health with the prospect of a higher rate of mortality as they experience a poorer quality of life.

We all grow older. The rate at which you age may not be obvious at age 20, when peak development stops, but as the years and decades go by, it becomes undeniable. However, the *rates* of change due to age are largely determined by your lifestyle, which then impacts health. Lifestyle includes many factors, such as diet and quality of sleep, your ability to deal with stress, and your resilience. Probably the greatest risk factor to a healthy active aging is a lifestyle featuring a lack of movement, specifically regarding how many hours you sit every day.

Studies show that 75 percent of persons over the age of 65 sit more than eight hours per day. To some extent this might be related to altered post-retirement habits and lifestyle. Perhaps a partner died or you are living alone for other reasons where the need to get up and do something for someone else has diminished or disappeared. Possibly you have moved in with younger family members and you no longer need to do household chores and yard work. You are encouraged to "take it easy," or your family might be worried that you could fall and break something.

At my talks, I encourage the audience to stand up, unassisted if at all possible. A very spry and upright 80-year-old member of my audience stood up quite easily. Yet at the end of the talk, I noticed that she used a walker. On probing, I discovered that she had moved in with her daughter's family, where there was a step down to the family room. As a precaution, she was forbidden to walk even in the house as well as outside without a walker. I suggested she stand up as often as possible, unassisted in a safe place, throughout the day to strengthen her legs, balance, and mostly her confidence. Then she could have the whole family take the aging-well test!

Debra Rose, director of the Aging Well Center in Fullerton, California, has developed a test to assess the level of incoming participants of the center. The test involves sitting upright in an armless chair, feet flat on the floor, arms crossed across the chest, and using a timer to measure how many times you can stand up straight-backed and unassisted in 30 seconds. It is a very discriminating test. Nine to 14 is average. If you can stand up over 24 times in 30 seconds, you are doing very well. Less than nine times means you need help badly. I find it useful to test myself if I want to intersperse an exercise in my day and as a reminder of how I am doing. A friend tells me the test/exercise is a great pick-me-up to renew energy every few hours. I recommend it to anyone, whatever your age.

I also meet many mature couples who sell their home and go to live in a retirement community, some in the "continuing care" style that offers assisted-living services if and when needed. At first, they participate in a range of activities, but depending on friends they may or may not make, interest wanes. They become more home-bound and sedentary.

One of the problems with advancing age is a pervasive dysfunction of small and large blood vessels that results in stiffening of the main central elastic arteries, increased blood pressure, and erosion of the endothelial lining of peripheral blood vessels. An ever-growing literature now supports the notion that these breaks in endothelium are crucial in the development of vascular diseases, like atherosclerosis and high blood pressure, and may also affect physical function. Separate from its effects on blood flow and tissue perfusion, NO (Nitric Oxide) in the endothelial lining also plays a significant role in optimally maintaining the skeletal muscles' ability to contract. It normally helps muscle fiber shorten faster in order to reach peak contraction with greater force. Conversely, reduced NO, as happens rapidly with sitting, even for as little as three hours, leads to reductions in muscular power and strength. The risk of adult-onset (Type 2) diabetes also increases with age. As Nir Barzilai and colleagues at the Albert Einstein College of Medicine in New York City wrote: "The aging process is charac-terized metabolically by insulin resistance, changes in body composition, and physiological declines in growth hormone (GH), insulin-like growth factor-1 (IGF-1), and sex steroids."[50] A sedentary lifestyle, again, contrib-utes to these problems.

The increase in sitting time in the elderly is the result of a vicious cycle—especially after retirement when, instead of filling that extra time with a job, volunteering, exercise classes, gardening, and household activities or meeting up with friends, it is easier to avoid doing anything until it becomes difficult or impossible to move at all. Worse still, a fall may cause a fracture, a setback from which it is hard to recover. Having to move out of your home is often the first step, the decision of where to move to is the second—whether with family or into a nursing facility.

I have visited and talked with residents of many such homes. The homes provide an extraordinary service. Most are clean, with kind, helpful, considerate staff, excellent meals, social groups, and even outings. But in most you cannot help feeling a helpless apathy toward the downward slide. The environment is emotionally sterile and there is far too much sitting. (In part this is because a sitting resident is safe from the risks of falling; they do not require as much attention or care.) Sitting is a form of sensory deprivation, creating a lack of touch and a lack of a variety of tastes, smells, and noises, other than the monotonous sound of TV. There is no changing scenery, little variation in the people seen each day, and hardly any human interaction and conversation. Lack of interest in anything and everything follows and likely leads to depression. From depression to dementia is a short step. Depriving your brain blood flow with sitting cannot help Alzheimer's disease, Parkinson's, or any other brain condition. For residents in a nursing home or retirement care facility, the TV is on all day and often serves merely as background noise. Why would anyone in a nursing home be interested in the lineup of moving mouths of an array of presidential hopefuls?

Some facilities are more creative. I spoke at the Doak Walker Care Center in Steamboat Springs, Colorado. The residents were housed next door to a preschool; once a day the small children came over to visit and interact. They made friends quickly and some bonding took place. The visit was highly anticipated; it was the highlight of everyone's day and friends were quickly made. Young and old looked forward excitedly to their daily visit, and it was a big emotional boost to both groups. Co-located nursing and preschooler facilities have successfully been in practice for quite a few years in Japan. Outdoor playgrounds for seniors have been built in Finland and Germany.

At a local nursing facility, I worked out a plan with the enthusiastic physiotherapist to get those who volunteered to join a "stand up every thirty minutes" activity as a means of regaining independence. We put our proposal in for review by management. Two weeks went by with no reaction. On further probing, I was in for an eye-opener, having been told: "For personal safety reasons they could not have participants stand up unassisted and there would not be enough available staff for one-on-one monitoring." Improving personal independence was not what the nursing home was about. Families who visit nursing home candidates for a loved one look at cleanliness, kindness of the staff, environment, meals, facilities, and care. They would never imagine the extent of the harmful inevitable effects of too much sitting and the emotional sensory deprivation of such an environment. It's a one-way road.

There are other possibilities, however. There are small, portable pedaling devices that may be useful in nursing homes to use while sitting watching TV, whether alone or in a group, to provide enough energy to stimulate circulation, and maybe have the chance to send some blood up to the head as well. Walkers are useful support for mobility, but most of those using them end up with stooped posture as they habitually stand over the device. Stooping comes with its own poor health consequences.

As I have mentioned earlier, the data we have on sitting does not reflect whether it is in large uninterrupted blocks of time, as I suspect. Add to that the cumulative decrease in the amount of moving about in the course of daily living and your rate of aging takes a nosedive. It all has to do with how much you use the gravity that surrounds you. Do not use it at your peril. Use it and you have the opportunity for a vibrant, dynamic life. How do we know that? It is quite simple. While living in almost no gravity in space, astronauts' bodies age at least 10 times faster than you age here on Earth. Muscles waste, bones lose their density and are more likely to break, and vision, balance, skin, sleep, and the immune system are impaired. Actually, there is no point listing every negative health consequence of living without gravity because absolutely everything goes south. Genetics play a role mostly by predetermining which body functions are most vulnerable and therefore most likely to show adverse effects first or to the greatest degree.

Look at the other side. Centenarians, those beyond the age of 100, in general are healthier than younger "old" persons because they have maintained an active, curious attitude and move all day long.

Exercise, however modest, was found to be progressively beneficial to the elderly. A large study[51] followed 120,000 individuals aged 63–73 for 13 years. A low dose of activity of just 15 minutes per day, even at that relatively late stage in their lives, reduced their rate of mortality by 22 percent. It does not take much. It is a matter of incorporating all-day activities in daily living.

PEOPLE WITH PARALYSIS AND RELATED CONDITIONS

Spinal cord injury (SCI), with its accompanying lower body paralysis, is a form of chronic forced sitting. Along with bed rest, it has served as a model of sedentary behavior resembling the experience of astronauts in space, as they essentially do not use their legs. Of course, astronauts return from space and can recover by walking about on Earth, but most individuals with spinal cord injury face severe limits on the extent of recovery that is possible for them. Nevertheless, what we know about gravity and its effects can be used to help these individuals and others who, for one reason or another, need to use a wheelchair for all or part of their daily mobility needs.

Those who need to use wheelchairs can still benefit from harnessing gravity to the extent that their bodies are able, or can become able, to do so. It used to be thought that paraplegics could not sit up because they had a tendency to faint when they tried to sit, so they spent their entire life in a supine position. Eventually, though, it was figured out that the problem was one of circulation (hypotension, a drop in blood pressure with the postural change of sitting up) rather than the result of their severed nerve supply. Thus, it became apparent that, just as in returning astronauts, this blood pressure drop could be prevented. The body perceives and reacts to this postural change all the same because the sensors that control this blood pressure response are above the point of spinal cord damage.

This discovery changed the lives of persons with SCI. Assuming that a good part of the head-ward stimulus is due to circulation, which remains intact, postural change signals from lying down to sitting up frequently continue to be beneficial. This holds true not only in individuals with spinal cord injury, but also for many with other conditions that make it a challenge to sit up, and even for "normal" healthy patients during post-surgery rehabilitation.

The next step for those with spinal cord injury was to exercise their upper body. Some of them can reach exceptional levels of strength and endurance through upper body physical exercise, though they must cope with forced physical inactivity due to lack of nerve stimulation of the lower body. Extraordinary athletes emerged in wheelchairs on cross-country runs, on the tennis and basketball courts, and even on ski slopes in specially designed chairs.

Creative technologies were the result. Organizations developed by Andrea and Craig Kennedy like Access Anything: I Can Do That! and Adaptive Adventures, working state by state, opened up endless possibilities for individuals with spinal cord injury and other motor disabilities to participate in stimulating activities like travel and sports. One promising invention is the StandUp Wheelchair made by The Standing Company (based in Michigan). Designed for those who cannot stand on their own, this wheelchair holds the person in an upright position. To change position at regular intervals, some persons may still require help, but by remaining upright for many hours per day they are gaining access through gravity's benefits to a vastly greater extent than they otherwise would. Now we may see some of them stand up as they check-out at the supermarket, reach a shelf that was not previously accessible, make a presentation at the office, or have a discussion with their boss eye to eye.

PART TWO

HOW TO ENJOY LIFELONG HEALTH THROUGH SMART AND FREQUENT MOVEMENT

Chapter 4

The Mechanism at Work that No One Told You About

Gravity is a force of the universe that holds planets and stars together. Our Earth rotates around itself and around the sun, exposing us to the sun's light for about half of the twenty-four hours it takes for each rotation. During the other half we are in darkness. Depending on what part of Earth we live on and the season, we experience longer or shorter periods of light and darkness. We have day and we have night. When it is dark, we lie down to sleep. When daylight comes, we wake up. It is time to get up and do things. We stand up, sit down, and move, going about the business of living. We move throughout the day until it is time again to lie down at night.

Born on an Earth surrounded by these forces, we had to adapt and evolve to be best suited to live in Earth's changing environment. In our case, as human bipeds, we had to learn to stand and move upright, reaching for the sun or the heavens or up a tree to pluck some fruit. Gravity's main purpose for us is to use it to challenge and stimulate our bodies from the time we are born, so that we can remain upright and become perfectly adjusted to living on Earth. If we do not use gravity, we are in trouble. We stoop, have trouble moving, lose our balance—we age faster and gravity drags us down. Understanding the significance of using gravity on Earth and learning to use it effectively could put off the ravages of aging that we previously thought inevitable.

OUR RELATIONSHIP TO GRAVITY

As long as we are living on Earth, we are exposed to Earth's gravitational force. As we are asleep or awake, day or night, in light or darkness, we experience various intensities of gravity. That is not because gravity changes. The force of gravity pulls in one direction only: downward towards the center of the Earth. And its force does not change. Scientists call it 1G. It is by how we orient ourselves towards this 1G and by how we move about in it that we can modify how much or how little of this force our body experiences.

Think of "pole dancing" when you want to understand how to use gravity. Pole dancing has become a well-known entertainment among patrons of bars and clubs. We could use the term in a more literal sense to describe the "dance" we all execute with gravity as we go about our daily lives. We can picture ourselves dancing around a virtual pole of gravity that draws us and everything else on Earth—dust, plants, animals—downward. It keeps us from floating off into the universe. As we dance around this pole of force, we can vary the intensity of the G we feel. When we stand up, we experience G in the downward head-to-toe direction. We call it the Gz vector, which denotes direction. Less Gz is felt when we sit because our vertical column is shorter and supported by a seat. When we lie down, we further reduce the Gz we feel to almost nothing, because we now feel its force across our chest. We still experience G, but the vector is changed relative to our body. We call this vector Gx, and it seems to have minimal physiological significance that we know of.

The single-direction force of G does not change. However, we vary the influence of the Gz vector on our body throughout the day by when and how we move during the entire day. In this way, we use Gz as an intermittent stimulus to keep our body systems primed and tuned so that they can remain responsive to any demands. For example, when we have to run away from something, our heart beats harder and faster to get our blood moving so that we provide our body with the energy resources it needs. The more we move, the more responsive this reaction becomes, so that the next time we need to move our heart does not have to work as hard to get to the same heart beat or rate. In the exercise world, we call this becoming fitter. Some think of it as sharpening one's reflexes, but it applies to everything about how our body works, not only for neural responses. This process of initiating a response as part of deliberate training, as controlled repetition, can be applied to every system in the body. I call it tuning.

Most of us are not conscious that this is what we're doing, so the first task is to bring what we do, our habits, to consciousness: become aware of how long we are spending in a sitting position, a standing position, sitting slouched or upright, and so on. To take advantage of what gravity has to offer, the best thing we can do is to cultivate a habit of moving up and down. For example, we can stand up and squat down, then raise ourselves back up again, as our ancestors did day in and day out, and as people in developing countries typically still do today as they go about their everyday activities.

As we move about, we hardly feel gravity because we have adapted to it. But this adaptation wears off when we reduce gravity's influence by lying down or sitting in Earth's 1Gz for a prolonged period or by being launched into space and exposing ourselves to an environment of microgravity that is below the minimum threshold needed to sense Gz. We feel the consequences when we stand up again or return to Earth. You know how that feels if you have been in bed for a few days with the flu or you are recovering from an injury: When you try to get up and go about your usual activities, you may feel a little weak, dizzy, or uncoordinated. Your heart has to beat harder to get your blood up to your head so that you do not pass out. Your bladder control may not be as strong as it previously was. Outer space, bed rest, and chair sitting all produce the same changes, which are the result of being deprived of gravity or minimizing its influence. So does aging, especially if we allow the aging process to take its course without making use of gravity's benefits. Once the effects of gravity deprivation have set in, if you want to live upright again, you have to relearn to live in Gz and adapt all over again.

Gravity is our friend and keeps us Earth-healthy, if only we use it. If you stop using gravity because you are physically unable or get lazy about how you use it by sitting too much and slouching, the consequences will be painful and unpleasant. Sitting without a break makes you sick—you know how you feel after sitting in an all-day business meeting with very few breaks. Now imagine how you would feel if forced to remain sitting for much longer, as has happened in some hostage situations. In such a case forced sitting can become akin to torture, just as forcing a child to sit can be punishment. In modern life, we seem to have forgotten the harm of prolonged sitting, something that traditional religions may have figured out centuries ago. Consider how many religious services involve alternations between standing, sitting, kneeling, bowing the head and straightening up—not to mention the array of postures that form the essence of an ancient religious practice that has become very popular in the West: yoga! The unpleasant health consequences of prolonged, uninterrupted sitting occur because we as a society have neglected to use gravity as it was meant to be used. Modern conveniences, appliances, and transport mechanisms have diverted the need to move during the daylight hours when we are awake and active. In today's sedentary society—at the office, in your car on the road, or in your home—you no longer need to move for essential natural activities. A body, like a piano if not used, gets out of tune. It does not respond to the pianist's touch. It does not perform the way it should.

Health issues follow. As discussed in Chapter 3, the list includes but is not limited to metabolic syndrome including Type II diabetes, obesity, cardiovascular disease, cancer, and immune disorders, as well as sleep, balance, emotional, and cognitive issues. For example, David Dunstan's research shows that 30 to 60 minutes of sitting leads to measurable changes in triglycerides and the processing of sugar that are early signs of metabolic disease. Equally, just one hour in bed can result in a woozy feeling when you stand up again, particularly if you are a person with normally low blood pressure, such as a fit athlete. Whether sitting causes all of these health issues is not unequivocally proven. However, 75 percent of Americans aged 50–70 sit more than eight hours a day. Charles Matthews of the National Cancer Institute and his international team reported that sitting more than seven hours a day was mostly associated with high mortality risk of all causes, and specifically with cardiovascular mortality, as compared to those who sat only one hour a day. Sitting more than 11 hours a day increased the risk of dying by any cause by 40 percent in men over 45 years of age. Many people now sit more hours than they sleep. There is ample evidence that a sedentary lifestyle makes all these conditions worse and increases mortality.

Gravity has determined how we evolved, develop, grow, look, and function. How we use gravity determines our health and longevity. The benign neglect that comes with too much sitting has taken away our health, our ability to move about easily, and our ability to retain a youthful life. Essentially, the input to our central nervous system that moving in G is designed to provide is reduced by sitting. When the vestibular system, the brain's G-perceiving balance center, goes silent or is damaged, the rest of the body atrophies and prepares metabolically to shut down. Similarly, the hydrostatic system that pushes fluids around the body slows down. Slower circulation means slower shear forces in the blood vessels, where the endothelium lining is weakened by not being stimulated. Oxygen and nutrients are not carried around to the places they are needed to nourish, including the brain, where brain blood flow is reduced, affecting how the brain works. The sense of weight load on muscles and bones is reduced, requiring lower energy needs and output. Lipoprotein lipase, the enzyme that mops up fats from the circulation, is reduced and muscle glucose is preserved by increased resistance to insulin. The sense of direction and acceleration is removed and there is no change in posture and position while you sit; the signal triggered by a change in posture mediated by the vestibular system goes silent. Balance and coordination are confused. This is akin to sensory deprivation, where what you are deprived of is the ability to sense gravity and direction. The overwhelming signal from sitting is that of self-preservation, as energy, metabolic activity, circulation, and all functions prepare to shut down. We have taken our hunter-gatherer ancestor and sat him in front of a computer.

HOW TO MAKE FRIENDS WITH GRAVITY

To take advantage of what gravity has to offer and maintain a healthy state, we need to restore this Gz neural input with repeated daily, all-day vestibular stimulation. Gz also works mechanically, pushing and pulling every single cell in the body either directly or indirectly as we move. The key to this stimulation is moving: Movement that specifically challenges the Gz vector is the secret cure to our sedentary modern life. This sounds so simple that it is difficult to accept. After all, nobody is stopping you from moving all day! But the fact is that we don't. The Centers for Disease Control found that 80 percent of Americans do not do enough moving or exercise on a regular basis.

Changing posture, as in alternating standing up and sitting down, is the most efficient single signal to give our body in making friends with gravity. Exercise, which many of us do when we go to the gym or go out jogging, merely puts energy demands on muscle without correcting the ongoing problem of inactivity. It may seem surprising if I tell you that exercise once a day is ineffective in countering the effects of prolonged sitting. After all, aren't we given to believe that exercise can cure everything from cardiovascular disease to depression? Exercising frequently during the day would help counteract sitting to a degree, but this would be because of the additional posture changes, not the exercise itself. Not only that, but standing up frequently would work, either with or without the exercise. These were my findings in 1992 during a series of bed-rest studies to determine what would prevent the consequences of lying in bed continuously for four days. Standing up 16 times a day (once every hour, except during eight hours of sleep) turned out to be consistently more effective than walking 16 times a day every hour for the same amount of time! I was as surprised as you might be.

At a dinner of the International Academy of Astronautics, I was honored with an award for my book *The G-Connection: Harness Gravity and Reverse Aging.*[3] After receiving it, I made my way back to my table in the dimmed lights when I was stopped by someone who asked, "What is your book about?" "How to stay young and healthy as long as you live," I answered. "Oh yes? How?" the man asked. Stupidly, because I had not noticed that he was in a wheelchair, I said, "Stand up every thirty minutes," and went briskly on my way back to my table. A young man at our table asked me about this conversation. "Do you know who that was?" No, I did not. "That was George Mueller. He is 92 years old." For anyone who knows their space history—as I certainly should, given my many years of working for NASA—they might remember that a very young George Mueller was known as "Mr. Apollo" when he was Apollo Project Manager. I was humbled and felt I could have been more considerate and forthcoming, but I soon forgot about the incident.

Three months later, I got a call from the young man at our table. "I wanted to tell you a remarkable story. We were invited to the Muellers for dinner, rang the doorbell, and to our amazement George answered and proceeded to serve drinks—no wheelchair, at least in their home!" On his asking Mrs. Mueller "how come?", the young man told me that she replied, "He did it all by himself." "Did what?" "Stood up every thirty minutes." Admittedly, I found it hard to believe—not that standing up would help, but that it would make such a dramatic difference in such a short time.

Since then I have had success with six more individuals, one woman and five men aged 73 to 92, regaining various degrees of mobility with this intermittent standing up approach. If you or someone you know has a mobility predicament, it is worth a try. Maintaining mobility is the most crucial single aspect of successful aging.

TUNING THE BODY

Every body function, and probably every cell in the body, fluctuates in a rhythmic manner. Whether the rhythm is a circadian one, like body temperature cycling through the night and day, or the frequent oscillations of brain electrical activity, the EEG, and sleep rhythms, heartbeat, blood rate and pressure, breathing, gastric motility, swallowing, blinking eyes, or the episodic pulsating secretion of hormones, they each fluctuate with a typical optimal frequency.

Most of us know that jet lag makes us feel awful. And we know that jet lag occurs when rhythms are thrown out of synch by time zone changes when we fly across the globe. But we may not have thought about the many kinds of rhythmic fluctuations in the body that I've just mentioned. It's not just a matter of getting a night's sleep, much less sleeping on the airplane; instead, we need to allow our many bodily systems to return to their optimal rhythms. All is well again when the synchrony of several rhythms are back in relation to each other and the environment is restored. We feel better and our health is restored when systems function in synchrony. It's like the music made by a good orchestra synchronized under the baton of a great conductor.

An out-of-tune body is an unhealthy body. Good car mechanics can listen to a car engine and tell if something is wrong. You can feel a well-maintained car run smoothly. The same is true for a well-maintained body. No amount of medicine can replace proper body tuning. Being well-tuned means that your body may respond at a second's notice in an emergency or when needed. Tuning the body's systems creates a lasting foundation of health that can be continually built upon. Gravity is your tuning fork. But, unlike your piano, you need to take your body to gravity for its tuning. Your body is a perpetual motion machine. Continuous movement in and out of gravity will keep you in tip-top tuned shape.

Answers are coming from studies on aging

My 99-year-old uncle Nicolas was crossing the street when he was hit by a car that jumped a red light. His femur in his upper leg was broken, but fortunately not his hip. He called me from his hospital bed to ask what he should do. My first reaction was to tell him to get out of the hospital as soon as he could. Realistically, I suggested that every 30 minutes he should sit up with his legs hanging over the side of the bed, then lie down again after a minute or two. Then, once he was back home again, I advised him to stand up once every 30 minutes. He did get out of the hospital the next day and followed my prescription. To the amazement of the orthopedic surgeon, his bone healed in two weeks.

In a study with older adults aged 65 to 94 who maintained low levels of physical activity that would not meet physical activity recommendations, Louis Sardinha at the University of Lisbon, Portugal, presents some important observations that raise new questions about the relative importance of physical activity and breaking up sitting time as intervention. Physical function in this context corresponded to their ability to perform normal everyday activities safely and independently, without undue fatigue. It shows that if older adults break up sitting time more often, they may in fact improve their poor physical function. They may unexpectedly experience better aerobic capacity, skeletal muscle performance, flexibility, agility, and dynamic balance—all attributes that are measures of physical function in the elderly. On the other hand, and quite surprisingly to many, adding moderate-to-vigorous physical activity for 30 minutes per day resulted in *lower* physical function. Clearly, with these subjects, breaking up sedentary time provided benefits that vigorous physical activity did not.[52]

TELOMERES KEEP US YOUNG

Another piece of significant relevant research came from a completely different perspective. The discovery of the role of telomeres in aging won Elizabeth Blackburn[53] at the University of California, San Francisco, a Nobel prize in Medicine in 2009. Telomeres are the tips of chromosomes in cells that divide. Their length tells us a lot about the host's health. Telomerase is the enzyme that influences the length of telomeres. Telomere length is a primary biomarker of cellular aging that has been associated with cardio-vascular disease, insulin resistance, hypertension, and mortality. With age, emotional stress, and various diseases, these telomeres shorten until they disappear and the cell dies. Malcolm Collins and his colleagues at the University of Cape Town, South Africa, found that athletes diagnosed with "fatigued athlete myopathic syndrome" (in other words, overdoing it) had shorter muscle telomere length than their age counterparts.[54] Adding to this concept, Lynn Cherkas and her group at King's College, London, found that more moderate leisure-time physical activity improved telomere length.[55] Moreover, the benefits increased in a dose-dependent manner— the more frequent was physical activity the longer were the telomeres. This research provided the first evidence of a role for typical physical activity in modifying telomere length.

Andrew Ludlow and coworkers at the University of Maryland studied the telomere length of men and women aged 50 to 70 in relationship to their level of activity. They divided their participants according to their exercise energy expenditure into four groups: 0–990, 991–2340, 2341–3540, and greater than 3540 kilocalories (Kcal) per week. They found no relation-ship between exercise intensity and telomere length. The second group of 991–2340 Kcal/week had significantly longer telomere lengths than either the lowest or the highest energy expenditure groups. These results indicate that moderate physical activity levels may provide a protective effect on blood mononuclear telomere length compared with both very low and very high exercise expenditure levels. There appears to be an optimal mid-level of activity for the greatest benefit to telomere length.[56]

In terms of assessing gravity's benefits, the message is that sedentary behavior should not be addressed as cumulative time spent sitting, which most meta-analysis studies have relied on. Instead, studies need to measure the length of time spent sitting before it is interrupted by the next change in posture. This time period, taken from Dr. David Dunstan's and my work,[28, 9] is somewhere around a maximum of one to two hours for minimum damage and less than 30 minutes for optimal health. How breaks in sedentary behavior act and how long of an optimal period spent upright is required at each break remain to be resolved.

INTERVENTIONS: WHAT WORKS AND WHAT DOESN'T

We need to correct misunderstandings about what interventions are best for us. Government recommendations as well as those from national health organizations like the National Heart Association have been so indoctrinated by the need to exercise that they rarely think or question what that means. Surely, it would seem less exercise, or rather less intense exercise, cannot be better? But who then asks the question, "Better for what"? There is no such thing as one-size-fits-all needs. Popular health magazines are replete with images of young muscular persons and exercise routines that imply you will look like the image by following some exercise regime that is claimed to work in the minimum amount of time, since there is always a premium on time (as well as effort) in our modern life. In today's fast-paced world, human physiology that evolved over millions of years is in a state of shock.

Sitting is a natural, indeed necessary, part of living, needed to interrupt moving. It is very difficult if not impossible to refrain from sitting altogether, given today's lifestyle. However, the good news is that there are some excellent strategies to help counter the effects of sitting—and they are not that difficult to learn and incorporate into your daily routine. What it takes is a little self-awareness and examination of our daily habits. So don't take this news sitting down!

There are some obvious solutions offered to the problems caused by sitting, though not all of them work as well as others:

- Standing
- Sitting less total time
- Exercise
- Interrupting sitting

What is it we do when we sit and what do we not do? To restore health, we need to maintain awareness of the many other things we could be doing rather than sitting. This awareness needs to grow into a habit, which in turn will remind us to structure our day into activities that introduce normal and pleasant movement naturally back into our day.

STANDING

Obviously, sitting is thought of as the opposite of standing. Therefore, the argument goes, instead of sitting, we should spend more time standing. As a result, a variety of ingenious standing options have been invented, such as desks with elevated shelves for computers and modified chairs designed for standing to perform tasks.

Anyone who works at a job that requires too much standing, as in security guard work, retail sales clerking, nursing, or some forms of factory work, will tell you that standing is a pain, literally. The problems that persistent standing generates are just as troublesome as, although different from, those of prolonged sitting: severe back pain, neck pain, sciatica, shoulder pain, foot problems, swollen feet, aching knees, circulation problems like blood clots, and possibly light-headedness with fainting spells. Prolonged static standing should be avoided as much as prolonged static sitting. What is different about standing is that for most of us, standing usually involves the freedom to walk about and to take sit-down breaks when our legs and feet get tired. Spontaneously moving about is more likely. Sitting, in contrast, can literally go on for hours. After cumulative sitting, it becomes harder to stand up without help. Clearly, both standing and sitting are essential elements of daily living. The issue is that modern society has swung the pendulum much too far in favor of sitting.

To restore standing to its rightful place in the continuum of human postures, a variety of technological solutions have been generated with mixed success. Manufacturers introduced standing desks, and treadmill desks were not far behind. However, treadmills offered no apparent added value, since aerobic exercise is now recognized as not being the missing link to correcting the ills of extended sitting. They are also bulky and expensive. I would find them distracting to work on. Various bicycle or pedaling devices have also been developed, and these may provide exercise that burns some calories, or even provide some short-term circulation benefit, but they are not helpful in counteracting sitting. Changing-level work stations have gained in popularity and many improvements have been made in the technology to make them lighter and more versatile. Assessments of their effectiveness have been few, but the concept is promising since it facilitates positional change. Those that have a seat that moves up to provide you with the ability to perch periodically while you stand show promise.

Studies show increased productivity, better respiration, reaction, and alertness when standing, as compared to sitting. Dr. Mark Benden at the Texas A & M ergonomics center has accumulated evidence that you burn more calories standing and many less sitting.[57] Whereas sitting decreases cognitive skills, standing improves cognition, which means better productivity; however, both taken to extreme result in mental fatigue after as little as 30 minutes and certainly after five hours. Standing reduces the impact of bad-back-sitting, though it also depends on how you stand. Slouched standing increases neck and back pain and creates problems for the legs and feet. These are relieved by using a footrest, which forces one to shift from one leg to the other, or by using an arm-level rest, such as those designed into standing desks for children. A tall stool to lean or perch on may also be incorporated. A variety of forced movement interrupts stationary standing and forces better circulation and also redistributes weight in a way that cannot be done while sitting.

Standing on a balance board while working at a stand-up desk has merits, but is just as distracting as the treadmill. What I find most useful is an adjustable board called the "active office board." About two inches high, it rests on foam square pads that can be moved closer or farther apart on Velcro straps to increase or reduce your sway. Instead of standing on the floor, the board provides slight motion, or none at all, adjusted to your abilities. It's enough to slightly stimulate balance and foot proprioceptors without distraction or causing you to lose your balance. Such slight motion would relieve back pain as well as foot pain. The desk may be adjusted to take into account the extra height.

A much lower-tech (and less expensive) approach is to boost people's awareness of how long they are sitting and how often they should take a stand-up break. In the workplace, employers can provide training to

71

increase awareness of the consequences of too much sitting as another aspect of encouraging employee participation in wellness programs. Any number of buzzers, alarms, or app-alerts can be used to signal that it is time to stand up.

A multicomponent approach was tested at the Baker IDI Heart and Diabetes Institute in Melbourne, Australia, involving 44 office workers and was successful in reducing workplace sitting time among 20- to 65-year-old workers.[28] The interventions tested included monitoring with activity devices, using height-adjustable workstations, staff education, manager emails to staff, management consultation, and face-to-face coaching with telephone support. Employees wore the monitors for seven days at baseline and for the next three months to the end of the study. They all worked an eight-hour day, of which they sat about 6.1 hours per day during the seven days before the testing time began. At the end of the three-month period, sitting time in the multicomponent group was reduced to a total of 4.30 hours per day and to 5.6 hours per day in the workstations-only group. Both groups saw sizable reductions in sitting time, though it is not clear if they sat in one block of time or broke it up and moved about during the day. These results are encouraging. The workstations seem generally acceptable and feasible. The more smoothly they move up and down the better. In this study, the workstation seems to have been the primary beneficial factor, with added benefits provided to a lesser extent by the degree of attention and reminders that added social and management interactions provided.

To advance the value of this type of workplace wellness program, the next step is to determine exactly how often the workers changed the level of their workstation and how long they remained standing upright. This information could be general or specific to each person. It could then be used to provide general feedback or specific feedback, tailored to the individual on their exact state of health at any time. Devices could be developed to buzz or alert when that health measure was exceeded.

Since it's unlikely that our civilization's love affair with technology will end any time soon, we are perhaps wise to envision a future in which technology helps us achieve our gravity goals. Such a future would include complementary technologies that combine detection with action. For instance, one complementary technology to a workstation would be to couple a StandDesk with the Darma pillow, designed to sense sitting duration as well as position. The pillow could also provide the alert via a smartphone app to encourage standing up. Another new technology called

SmartMove relies on a shoe insole that tracks the wearer's movements. As he or she moves, a small person on the TV screen imitates his movements, reflecting his actions. The insole, which can be fitted into any shoe, contains two sensors that can tell if a person is sitting, standing, walking, running, or cycling. Data collected from pressure and distribution is transferred to an application on an iPhone that can tell the user how much of their day has been spent active in each category. It will also send users a text alert if they have been sedentary too long. SmartMove is also planning a subscription-based trainer for users, customizing feedback for each individual user.

Sitting less total time

In looking for solutions to the adverse effects of sitting, most of the focus has been on sitting fewer hours per day. Studies have generally asked participants to recall total time spent sitting, so the answers are likely to be inexact and quite possibly inaccurate. Only occasionally has time spent sitting been monitored with an accelerometer. In contrast to pedometers that measure the steps you take, accelerometers sense changes in direction and sometimes speed as well. Direction and acceleration are features of our environment that we sense through the vestibular system in our inner ear that monitors balance, and therefore accelerometers provide you not only with your motion in one direction but also with aspects of more complex movement such as when you stand up.

Most researchers conducting studies looking into what constitutes the least amount of sitting time to cause changes have been surprised to find how quickly adverse changes can occur. Saurabh Thosar and colleagues saw clear evidence of dysfunction of the endothelial lining of blood vessels with 50 percent less dilation and lower rate of blood flow after just one hour of sitting, though things got worse after three hours.[23] Australian David Dunstan and his group found that even 30 minutes of sitting could trigger an increase in blood triglycerides.[28] This is indicative of the pre-diabetic response known as insulin resistance—the lesser ability of muscle to respond to insulin by taking up from the blood stream the glucose it needs to contract; thus, more insulin is required to provide the muscle with enough glucose. Dunstan believes that it all relates to muscles having to contract to maintain upright posture. "This small increase is equivalent to a 13 percent increase, which sounds very small, but the amount of energy expenditure gained would be roughly equivalent to a 45-minute brisk walk." There is no doubt that the muscle contraction involved has unarguable benefits. But is that the whole story? Is that all that is needed to counteract the effects of sitting? Or would the same contraction while remaining seated be just as good? Could you just sit at your desk with no ill effects merely by maintaining muscle contractions and energy expenditure? The research to answer that question has yet to be done. However, considerable evidence suggests that changing posture is an essential component to counteracting the ill effects of sitting.

Many more changes happen when you move, especially moving up and down, not least the effects on circulation. When you sit for a while you know that your ankles might swell as the blood pools to your feet and your heart does not have to pump as hard. The result is less blood reaches your brain. The brain relies on this blood flow to provide it with oxygen and glucose, which it does not make and needs to be supplied with in order to remain healthy and working. The first thing that happens when you stand up is that things get worse before they get better. The blood rushes even more to your feet, further draining the blood from your brain. To correct this brain drain, the heart and circulation instantly react. Increased cardiac output and stroke volume, as well as expanding blood volume, pump blood up to your brain to correct the drop in brain blood flow and resupply the brain cells with oxygen. This is why standing up often helps your brain cells function better. However, the longer you stand still, the more gravity will pull blood back to your feet, your ankles will swell once more, and the increased brain blood flow cannot be maintained unless you keep moving up and down. It may help to shift your weight from leg to leg or contract the big leg muscles as the guards do in front of Buckingham Palace. Brain blood flow will not increase much, though, unless you do something more energetic like stomping your feet or taking steps and coming to attention. The increase in brain blood tissue oxygenation that follow standing coincides with improvements in cognitive abilities. These benefits are decreased during prolonged sitting, as has been observed by Stuart Biddle at Victoria University in Australia (2016). Awareness of how your body reacts to sitting and moving will guide you to what you need to do to keep your brain functioning as long as you live.

EXERCISE

It is obvious that sitting results in inactivity. Therefore, activity or exercise would logically be the solution to hours of sitting. Correct? It is well known that endurance exercise is important in reducing your overall cardiovascular risk as well as improving your fitness level. Exercise has been found useful in reducing symptoms of depression. Moderate to vigorous intensity exercise has been consistently associated with reduced risk of premature death. Exercise has been recommended to improve the ability to cope with the side effects of cancer treatment. It was therefore most surprising when direct comparisons were finally done, using different levels and types of activity, that what we think of as exercise—structured, once-a-day, fairly vigorous exercise—was ineffective or less effective than mild to low level activity in counteracting the ill effects of prolonged sitting.

Evidence is gradually appearing that interrupting sitting by getting off the couch neutralizes the effects of prolonged sitting. Veerman notes that "exercise is good but even light physical activity also improves health."[16] Similarly, Dunstan's group in Australia showed that light or moderate exercise for two minutes to interrupt sitting every 20 minutes was equally beneficial when measured using cardiometabolic markers.[19]

Several ongoing studies are accumulating evidence that exercise is not the panacea to the problems of too much sitting. However, light physical activity may have added benefits that might be unrelated to sitting. The issue is that individuals who exercise regularly and are physically fit come home eager to sit down and rest and probably eat because they are hungry. Despite their fitness, they respond to too much sitting just like anyone. Marc Hamilton, while he was at the Pennington Biomedical research center in Baton Rouge, Louisiana, said it clearly: "Sitting too much is not the same as exercising too little." In his group's studies, one hour of vigorous exercise daily did not compensate for the effects of sitting the rest of the day on insulin and blood lipids, both risk factors for diabetes and heart conditions.[8]

Measuring changes in muscle collagen, a marker of muscle function, Nielsen and associates found that the atrophy resulting from lying in bed continuously (bed rest) for 90 days was not prevented by daily resistive exercise when done in bed.[59]

INTERRUPTING SITTING

Interrupting sitting is the secret potion to health. It implies standing up as the first step to moving. Since in most cases any exercise condition by default begins with standing up, any study that evaluates the effect of exercise on sitting should be compared to a control that includes standing up only, without any exercise. As far as I am aware, no study has thus far incorporated such a control group in evaluating the benefits of exercise. So it is no surprise that all interventions that show benefit—interrupting sitting by standing up, vigorous exercise or mild to vigorous exercise—start off with standing up as a common factor. Exercise in the horizontal position during bed-rest studies (lying in bed continuously twenty-four hours a day) has been less than completely effective. Nor, to my knowledge, is there any evidence of a dose-response relationship—in other words, there is no study that shows that exercise is progressively more effective in counteracting sitting as it becomes more intense and/or is of greater duration. I am also unaware of any studies that explore short bouts of exercise throughout the day or studies that include for comparison a group that only stood up without moving.

In my 1992 study[9] exploring the benefits of standing or standing and walking at three mph on a treadmill every hour in preventing the consequences of lying in bed continuously for four days, I did include the standing-up-only group as such a control. I fully anticipated that standing up, without any exercise, would have no effect. Imagine my surprise when the results showed that standing was *more* effective than walking on a treadmill for the same length of time! Therefore, when sedentary health discussions began to gain steam, it seemed obvious to me that the change in posture element of standing up was likely more effective than any added exercise. However, the field in general was concentrating on calories and energy, favoring the focus on exercise as the logical answer to the ills of sitting. The results do not support it. It has now come full circle.

Bethany Barone Gibbs' team at the University of Pittsburgh used accelerometers to track the activity of 2,000 30- to 50-year-olds, for a week before and again after a five-year period to assess the odds of getting metabolic disease—the cluster of conditions that include high blood pressure and sugar levels, excess body fat around the waist, and abnormal fat metabolism markers that together are markers of the risk of serious disease, such as stroke, heart disease, and diabetes. Those who sat the longest every day, some for nearly 10 hours per day, were four times more likely to become diabetic five years later. She concludes:

> We are beginning to believe that being sedentary is something different than not getting exercise . . . Someone who runs 30 minutes every day can sit for the other 15 hours of their day at work, commuting and at home and this person would be considered physically active but also quite sedentary. On the other hand, a cleaning professional might never exercise but might spend most of their day on their feet in light activity—this person would be inactive but have very little sedentary time.[60]

Peter Katzmarik, who is affiliated with the Pennington Biomedical Research Center in Baton Rouge, Louisiana, agrees: "The results add to a growing body of evidence that even after you account for physical activity levels of these people, the amount of time spent being sedentary is positively associated with diabetic risk."[17]

Study after study now suggests that decreasing how many hours you sit continuously every day may be more closely linked to the occurrence of cardiovascular disease. As Cornell University scientist Rebecca Seguin says: "The assumption has been that if you're fit and physically active, that will protect you, even if you spend a huge amount of time sitting each day. In fact, in doing so you are far less protected from negative health effects of being sedentary than you realize."[47] Her research, one of the largest and most ethnically diverse of its type, finds that more everyday movement on top of exercise is also important for maintaining health. She emphasizes that small changes, like moving around inside and outside the house, make a big difference.

Catherine Falconer and her colleagues at the University of Bristol, UK, compared interrupting sitting with vigorous versus light to moderate physical activity. They concluded that even merely interrupting sitting time could improve the health of Type 2 diabetics as measured by lower BMIs, waist circumference, and higher HDL levels. "When the researchers analyzed how much the adults' metabolic health could improve with the different levels of activity, they found that HDL ('good') cholesterol rose with light physical exercise, though not with more vigorous exercise."[61] That runs counter to previous concepts.

Similar conclusions were drawn by Henson and associates at the University of Leicester that not only is sitting time strongly and adversely associated with cardiometabolic health in Type 2 diabetics, but breaks in sedentary time, as well as moderate physical activity, were beneficial.[62]

"I think the message that we don't even have to push for the moderate-to-vigorous physical activity, that breaking up your sitting time has demonstrable benefits, is actually pretty compelling," said Dr. Eddie Phillips, who founded and directs the Joslin Diabetes Center's Institute of Lifestyle Medicine in Boston. Dr. Phillips went on to comment that:

> It is a valid criticism to say we have not convinced the public to walk more appreciably, and those recommendations will remain, but if we can now recommend to patients that, "Jeez, if you just get up out of your chair

when the commercial comes on or drink more water and have to go to the bathroom," even that is enough to break up the prolonged sedentary bouts they describe in the research . . . . Breaking up sitting: Motivating people to spend less time in their chairs isn't easy, especially for those who work sedentary jobs at an office desk. Even people who meet the government's exercise guidelines may spend most of the rest of their days parked on a sofa or chair.[63]

Peter Kazmaryk adds:

You can start by getting up from your chair intermittently at work. Take walks around the hall in your office or try holding walking meetings instead of sitting around a table. Get up to chat with your colleague instead of sending an email. Standing doesn't take the place of exercise, but it should replace a good chunk of time you spend in your chair. The key is to spend as little time as possible sitting down.[18]

Not all sitting is equally bad

Interrupting sitting may be a powerful solution, but there is more to the sitting problem than just plain sitting for too long. How we sit also makes a difference. Poor static posture, even if you break it up and return spontaneously to that poor posture when you sit again, results in cumulative trauma, occlusions, and blockages of normal body flow and functioning that lead to pathology. Poor posture and being sedentary are affecting health nationally.

Consider how the downward pull of gravity enters and leaves your body. Is it through the back of your 15-pound head, pulling it down, past the front of your body and abdomen toward your pubic region? Giving in to this gravitational pull without engaging the muscles that hold the body upright will result in a slumping, slouched posture. Remember what your mom said at the dinner table: "Sit up straight, with elbows off the table." Now kids sprawl over the table, leaning on an arm that sometimes also holds up their head while eating.

When we slouch, we are collapsing the normal curve of the spine, forcing the spine and rib cage into an unnatural contortion, and running the risk of causing aches and pains from head to toe. Sitting with shoulders scrunched up will tighten the neck muscles, resulting in headaches, neck pain, and/or shoulder pain. The internal organs may be compressed, inter-

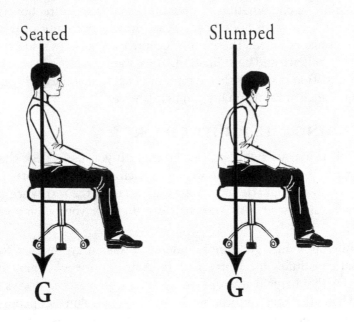

Figure 3. Correct (left) and incorrect (right) seated working posture.

fering with healthy breathing and blood circulation. A habitually hunched back can contract the wrong muscles and, over time, bring on a stooping stance that makes you look older than you are. Poor sitting posture may not only physically contort your body but also affect its relationship to the Gz vector, which in turn impacts your vestibular system, not to mention brain blood flow and function. Elementary school children stooped over some texting device for hours on end are now a common sight, this occurring at a time in development when the spine and skeleton in general is still developing. Will the next generation, as they become adults, have a curved spine with all its associated conditions, predominantly pain?

Do your feet hurt when you get out of bed in the morning? It might be the shoes you wear, but more likely it is the removal of proprioceptive stimuli to those soles as you sit. Both astronauts and bed-rest volunteers complain of painful foot soles when first stepping on firm ground again. After almost a year in space, Scott Kelly complained of such pain as well as pain in his joints and extreme sensitivity to anything that touched his skin. For those sitting at an office desk, some have suggested exercise by pedaling a compact bicycle beneath the desk, but this will not provide the required stimulus—a combination of pressure, weight, and direction (where your feet are relative to your head)—that gravity normally provides to keep those sensors tuned. These proprioceptive sensors are also crucial cues to proper balance and coordination. Thus, the premature loss of balance and coordination is yet another symptom of aging that becoming aware of the importance of using gravity can help prevent.

FINDING THE RIGHT CHAIR

This brings us right back to the chair. If you use a desk chair built for support, it may be just the wrong medicine, as its "support" is depriving you of normal muscle tone. Your muscles need the resistance provided by moving against gravity—no chair can do it for you when you are sitting still.

Attending an ergonomics conference was an eye-opener for me as to what constitutes the "correct" desk chair. "You would think twice about buying that bargain at your favorite office supply store,"[64] says Rani Luder of Humanics Ergonomics, Inc. In an office, "we don't let people move and we feed them a lot,"[65] says Jerome Congleton at Texas A & M. Employers generally buy office chairs in bulk; they are probably standard chairs designed for an "average" body. Since no one's body is actually "average," everybody is uncomfortable, everyone hurts. In my view, the simplest, healthiest solution is a hard-backed wooden chair with no arm rests. You may always add a small pillow.

THE EYES LEAD THE BODY

If you are a dog training enthusiast, you may have learned that the dog's nose leads the body: If you want the dog to sit, raise the nose and the hind-quarters will naturally lower to the floor. Humans are not too different. Did you know that your eyes lead your body? Optometrist Jeffrey Anshel, a vision consultant in Florida, is a leading expert in the study of eye health and your physical relationship to your computer. Dr. Anshel advises that when looking straight forward your eye level should be at the top of your screen. In that position your eyes can only be slightly downcast when you read, sparing both your eyes and your neck from strain. The height of your keyboard is equally important, with the optimal position being at a level that casting your eyes down to see it will not require bending your neck.

Once you have adjusted these, you can figure out where your arms and hands should be to avoid further strain. A little attention to this setup, at which most of us spend quite a lot of our time, can prevent a great deal of pain and injury and make healthy posture more natural.[66]

The other common situation where eyes and posture mesh together is when we sit or recline, sometimes for hours, to watch TV. According to what you have already read, you can, of course, predict that I advise standing up during each commercial break. Beyond that, consider the type of chair or sofa you are using, and how you are using it. If you're twisting yourself sideways because the TV is off to the side of the room, you obviously are not doing yourself any favors. Ditto if you are stretched out reclining on one elbow to peer up at the screen. It may not seem "relaxing" to sit up in a firm chair with your back straight and eyes straight ahead, but slouching through your favorite programs in a soft, comfy chair is asking for trouble, especially if you happen to take a nap in that position. Because you were neither lying down nor sitting correctly, you may feel awful when you wake up and wonder why. And do not succumb to the thought of buying a padded recliner chair that at the push of a button can raise you upright. Any time you get a device to do something for you, or as the advertising gurus say "to make your life easier," you are, in fact, signing your death warrant. You are not meant to sit endless hours. You are indeed designed to move.

THE J-CURVE AND THE CAMERA

Most of us who live in industrialized cultures have less than ideal posture. Esther Gockhale in Silicon Valley, California, has made a lifetime study of what is proper posture. By studying people's posture around the world, she came to the conclusion that ideal posture has a "J curve," as seen in many native peoples, in contrast to the "S curve" typically seen in Western societies. She describes steps to a good posture in her book, *8 Steps to a Pain-Free Back*. The bottom part of the "J" corresponds to your behind slanting out behind you, just as children stand with a straight back, lumbar area remaining relatively flat, with their bottoms out behind them.[67]

Now that you know what a healthy sitting posture looks like, observe how you sit. Freeze. Turn your camera on and look at yourself once a day to see how you are doing.

- Are both your feet flat on the floor?

- Are your legs tucked under you or bent at a 90-degree angle with your knees above your ankles?

- Are your abdominal muscles gently pulled in?

- Is your spine straight, leaning slightly back?

- Are your shoulders pulled down, your neck long, and your chest facing upwards?

- Is your chin parallel to the floor?

- Is the top of your head moving away from your shoulders, reaching up toward the ceiling?

Your goal is to sit, stand, and walk so that your blood flows freely, your back is supported, you breathe freely all the way down to your abdomen, and your body is aligned with gravity. If you are sitting in a healthy way, you will have a relaxed back and shoulders. You won't be giving yourself back or neck pain—and, better yet, you'll be less likely to "shrink" in height as you get older.

Healthy posture, both sitting and standing, pays off in additional ways. How you hold yourself matters. According to psychologists Li Huang and Adam Galinsky at Northwestern University, it can even boost your self-esteem and the admiration you receive from others.[68] Harvard Business School professor Amy Cuddy calls it a "power pose." She claims "standing like a superhero for just two minutes before a big challenge can provide a surge of confidence. How you hold yourself affects how you view yourself."[69]

To build a habit of good posture, become aware, wherever you are, of your posture while standing, sitting, walking. You may adapt it to your specific lifestyle and conditions. Your posture has a lifetime of benefits and is free. It actually pays you back through increased productivity, energy, state of mind, and lower health care costs—not to mention making you look more attractive and powerful. It is a small effort for a huge return.

Chapter 5

The Solution: Healthy Habits that Keep You Moving

A PLAN TO REVERSE SITTING'S DAMAGE AND PROTECT YOUR HEALTH

Sitting is as natural a part of living as standing up, sleeping, eating, and moving. It is physiological. Sitting only became pathological after its role in our modern daily life changed. The way we work has shifted, and the way we use our leisure hours is more sedentary. Instead of alternating between standing and moving, distributed evenly throughout the day, we now sit for a greater block of time and overall proportion of time than previously. This has resulted in making us less resilient, which damages our health while increasing the long-term risk of illness.

The solution to this mess involves actively confronting the problem. No pill, exercise device, or a new chair can do it for us. We need to refocus our awareness; we need to be selfish. We need to move more so that our cells are subjected to stimulating sensations as we move in the field of gravity. Yet it is not just any kind of G-moving. If there is a word that defines the solution to our sitting woes, it is *alternating*—from sitting to standing, from standing to bending over to pick something off the floor, from squatting to jumping up, from stretching up to bending sideways, moving up every which way, kneeling down in prayer to touch your forehead on the ground and back upright again. Add *frequent* and *variety* to *alternating* and you have the keys to the solution.

HOW YOU SIT AND MOVE

There is another part to sitting, apart from the sheer number of hours spent sitting. All movement is G-related movement, but the most valuable is that which is aligned with gravity in the head-to-toe direction, Gz. Alternate often into a standing position and you'll keep your vestibular system and your body tuned, with each change in posture moving blood up to your head. "A sure way to clear their head and improve their mood," says Dr. Eric Peper, professor at San Francisco State University, of his students when he asks them to stand up halfway through his classes. Yes, you can increase brain blood flow with your daily exercise routine, but that is only one time each day and it takes a lot of work to do it.

What we want to do is tap into a virtuous cycle based on each person's starting point and begin to move more frequently and more effectively. As you do this, I guarantee your levels of energy and strength will begin to increase, your confidence will be raised, and you will start to seek out opportunities to move more. This is the Golden Egg. Unless you are in a coma, you can move. You may suffer from a disability or be handicapped by obesity or age, but there is always *something* you can do.

HENRY HAD A STROKE

Henry, a 57-year-old man who had suffered a stroke seven years earlier, was in a wheelchair at one of my talks. The stroke had paralyzed his left arm, which was in a sling to get it out of the way. Otherwise, he seemed fine. He told me he had been an athlete. Now his sister solicitously tended to him. I asked if he could get out of his chair at all to use the bathroom. His sister said he could. I said, "Show us. Get up any which way you can." With some difficulty he struggled and succeeded to get up with this huge grin on his face. The audience burst out in standing applause as he stood there for a while relishing the moment, as his worried sister looked on. If he could walk, he could get around . . . and maybe even drive. He promised that he would continue to practice to strengthen his legs. It gave him new hope. A new life.

My experience with several even older persons has been that they can make real progress within three months if they make a habit of standing up every 30 minutes throughout the day. It does not have to be exactly 30 minutes. Twenty or even ten minutes will do or you may vary the times. It won't do to stand up every ten minutes for a block of time and then sit the rest of the time. The key is not to sit longer than 30 minutes at any one time. Men are more successful at this because they are more motivated to stick with the routine by the thought of regaining some degree of independence.

What we are trying to achieve here is to help you develop conditions that will encourage you to move ever more effectively. Visualize a common setting where you do a great deal of sitting, perhaps at work or at home on the sofa. Now visualize yourself standing up and moving, developing small habits that compel you to frequently change your posture. You have a powerful motivation: the freedom that comes with movement. Maybe you have decided you no longer want to rely on a wheelchair or a walker or you want to prove a point to someone else or to yourself that you can actually get out of your chair again and maneuver by yourself. There is hope.

Even if you are not wheelchair-bound but recognize that your muscles are getting weaker, this is a great routine to make them stronger. What's more, though this applies to people of any age, you can use Professor Debbie Rose's evaluation test designed at the University of California in Fullerton, Center for Successful Aging. On registering at her center she evaluates a patient's starting level by how many times he or she can stand up and sit down from a straight-backed chair in 30 seconds. The average is standing up nine to 14 times. More is obviously better. Less than nine times needs work.

Ultimately, we're talking about a shift in mindset from looking at exercise as the only savior to understanding and relishing that simply changing one's posture along the G axis and moving in more effective ways will create the foundation for your health.

Let's get moving!

MOVEMENTS YOU CAN DO AT HOME

WAKING UP

When you wake up in the morning, before you turn on your smartphone and while still in bed, take some slow deep breaths, grateful for the new day, and prepare to move.

- Remove your pillow in order to lie flat on your back.

- Rotate your hands and feet several times in both directions.

- Press your palms flat against each other and feel your arm muscles contract while you continue to press to the slow count of 10.

- Interlace your fingers and repeat, pressing and squeezing your fingers against your hands.

- Rotate your wrists again.

- Stretch your arms and legs in opposite directions, pointing fingers and toes as far away from each other as you can. Enjoy the stretch.
- Now bend your knees and lower them to the left. Feel the stretch up your right side as you hold the position.
- Repeat the stretch to the right.

Getting up

- Sit up. Slowly feel your feet on the floor and stand up—or do this next move sitting if you cannot stand up. I do this as often as I can even while sitting at my desk.
- Stretch up your arms again.
- Lean slightly to the left, pulling your right arm overhead with your left hand while pushing out into your right side.
- Then do the same, pulling the left arm to your right side.

Sitting exercise

Here is a special move you can do when sitting to release your back muscles, since when we first sit up or stand up the vertebrae in our spine are pulled down by gravity and collapse on each other. These muscles keep us tall as we age and prevent back pain.

- Begin by sitting up straight, looking straight ahead.
- Raise your head up. Obviously, your chest goes up, not your shoulders, your head goes slightly back in line with your chest (dropping it back is not good for your neck); your upper back arches backward as you pull your shoulders down.
- Enjoy the stretch.
- Then slowly droop your head forward to touch your chest with your chin, arch your back like a cat, bringing your shoulders in and down as if to meet each other.
- Feel the stretch between your shoulder blades and down the back of your neck.

Now you are ready to start the day.

WHILE WATCHING TV

The timing of TV commercials is a perfect opportunity for you to stand. Any time you watch TV, stand up during every commercial. They usually come up every 20 minutes and last for two or three minutes.

- Stand, go do something, or just sit down again when your program resumes.
- Fold the laundry or do your ironing while watching TV.

Not only does a stand-up break help keep your body well, but it spares your mind from the inane advertising exposure.

HOUSEWORK

- Cook actual meals ahead of time; they are healthier and tastier and you do not need to order pizza.
- Get out of the house if you have a garden; there is always a weed that needs picking. Growing your own garden is a terrific way to stay active.
- Anytime is also a good time for light housecleaning, dusting, and maintenance.
- Wash or wax your car yourself.
- Take your dog for a walk. If you did so earlier, take him or her out again.

MOVEMENTS YOU CAN DO IN YOUR CAR

Most of us spend a long time, sometimes hours, in our cars or on some other form of transportation. Short of getting out of the car to gas up in the middle of a commute (instead of before you set out), you can use the time while sitting to work on your core muscles.

- Make sure you sit up straight with shoulders pushed down.
- At traffic lights, suck your stomach muscles in and out as often as you can—it does wonders.
- If another driver's driving irritates you, relax by pushing your shoulders down, sitting up straight, and taking some slow deep breaths and a strong slow exhale to dissipate the stress.

- At a traffic light, turn your torso (not your head) slowly from the waist as far back as you can go, then turn your head as well. Wait for the next traffic light to turn in the other direction.

- Why drive at all? Walk and or take public transit even one day a week.

There are many obstacles we can conjure to breaking up our sitting: "I have a 75-minute commute each way, and a sedentary job where they want me planted to my chair." What would you do to introduce moving in your day? Opportunities exist, so be creative!

MOVEMENTS YOU CAN DO IN YOUR WORKPLACE

AROUND THE OFFICE

- Remember to stand up often during the workday.

- Stand up during meetings.

- Have meetings with your colleagues in person instead of relying on email. You can set a fixed time and get more accomplished than sitting in an office or cubicle. Even better, have standing and walking meetings, which are fast and efficient.

- Volunteer to stand up and get something for others.

- Don't stare at your smartphone while walking—you'll get "text neck."

- Take the stairs instead of the elevator whenever you can.

Back-up astronaut Bob Phillips used to take the stairs—seven flights up and down—at the NASA headquarters building in Washington, D.C. He said he got started doing so because he was fed up waiting for elevators. Sometimes, especially in the morning, he enjoyed the climb without having to listen to someone complaining about something first thing in the morning.

AT YOUR DESK

- Use any excuse to stand up often if you are working at your computer.

- Even while in your chair, it is important to maintain good posture between times when you stand up.

- Do some movements that open your shoulders, stretch your neck, and strengthen your arms and legs.

- Upward stretching and cat-cows work well, or just slide your elbows back and hold them there for a minute. Do you feel the relief of tension between your shoulder blades? This movement works your chest muscles in the process.

- Do half of a stand-up, stretching your arms overhead, holding one wrist at a time and leaning slightly sideways to stretch each side in turn, just as you did before getting out of bed in the morning. It's not quite like actually standing up, but any movement away from the ground challenges gravity and benefits you.

- What about your legs? While sitting in your chair with feet flat on the ground—this does not work well with stiletto heels—contract your thighs and push your feet into the ground as if to raise yourself off your seat. Hold the position as long as you can and release. This does wonders for the G-sensing proprioceptors in your bottom. Repeat as many times throughout the day as you think of it.

LUNCHES, BREAKS, AND MEETINGS

- If you make a habit of eating at your desk, change your habit or get up and join someone for a stand-up lunch.

- Are there people in your office or workplace who feel free to settle in a chair to chat while you are trying to work? You cannot shut the door to cubicles. Instead, organize short, working, walking meetings during the day, preferably outdoors. If someone wants to meet with you, take them out for a walk around the block. If they are not serious and just wanted to waste your time, they will soon learn not to do it again. Word gets around.

- If you are in a wheelchair, have workplace colleagues wheel you around the corridors or outdoors.

- If you work at home—we all do to some degree—take a walk with friends instead of always meeting for lunch to eat or drink while sitting. *Change your habits.*

MOVEMENTS YOU CAN DO AT SCHOOL

- If you teach, work at a school, or have school-age children, talk to them as well as to the teaching staff about the dangers of too much sitting.

- Set up situations to encourage standing up often, if only to change position. Sitting on the floor gives students reason to stand up. Sitting on a stool discourages sprawling on a desk or table and makes it harder to slouch but easier to stand up. Find a way of making smart movements desirable or rewarding.

- Call students up to a whiteboard or to the front of the class to explain something to the others.

- Create frequent opportunities for students to move, so their vestibular systems are stimulated. This will lead to better balance and improved attention and learning in the classroom.

- Organize frequent short or longer recesses and playtimes.

Since this is not something parents can control, instead encourage your child to go to school early whenever possible and play with friends. Arrange with some other parent for their children to arrive early at school as well to participate together with your children.

GET MORE PLAYFUL

Think back to when you were a child. Or watch a toddler at play. What was your idea of fun? How did you move and play? Did you climb up trees? Tumble? Jump rope? Your first bicycle? Hang upside down on monkey bars? Seventy-some-year-old Stephen Jepson in Florida has made it his life's work to reintroduce play into our lives. He is the best customer at Toys "R" Us. Invited all over the world, he travels with his toys, juggling, balancing on a bar, rollerblading, reminding us all of the fun we could have if only we allowed ourselves to be a child again. Age is no limit. Allow children to be a wonderful reminder to you!

WAYS I BREAK UP SITTING

I must confess that I do lapse in my standing up from time to time. I had to meet a tight deadline for a chapter (yes, on sitting behavior and health!) and it felt like I sat continuously for two weeks to get it done. I felt awful at the end of it, but I got it done! However, normally:

- I try to stand up about every 20–30 minutes.

- I avoid sitting in soft armchairs or on sofas when I am not working.

- When watching TV, I'm in the habit of getting up during commercials.

- I do something in the kitchen: I put something out to thaw, cook at night for the next day, or do mindless things that take only a few minutes and require or can be done standing up, like record-keeping or paying bills. I change into my pajamas, write in my diary, brush my teeth, put on some cold cream, set out pills for the next day, put out the garbage or whatever needs doing. Instead of doing it all at the same time, I deliberately spread it out.

- I make myself a cup of hot tea or just hot water on a cold day or cold mint tea on a hot day. I do not care for drinking water but quite like hot water either flavored with some ginger or with a few drops of hot sauce! Great in the winter.

- It also means I have to get up to empty my bladder every so often. This keeps me hydrated. Drinking small amounts throughout the day is better for hydration.

- I keep my printer more than arm's length away.

- My landline phone is five feet away. So I must get up to catch it before the answering machine comes on (which for some reason irritates me).

- My notes are on a table behind me, so I have to get up to reach them.

- I go to the window to stretch, arms overhead.

- I put a load of clothes into the wash. Usually the cycle of washing or drier is about 30 minutes and it buzzes when ready.

- My desk is next to the window. I see some bush or twig or weed needs to be trimmed or picked, plant watered, fallen leaves in the fall or snow path cleared. Doing this in small jobs rather than all at once is less tiring.

- I may go for a short walk to the top of the hill and back. It takes only 10 minutes.

The bottom line is that by staying active, moving, and connected, my reward is having energy all day, sleeping well at night, feeling healthy, and being happy and fulfilled.

Chapter 6

The Plan: 8 Key Steps to Enjoying Lifelong Health

This chapter explores eight ways to move smartly, using gravity—starting right now!

1. Move in the line of gravity

This is simply about standing up without going anywhere. A change in your posture is the most crucial signal to body health and the single smartest movement you can do.

As Yoga therapist Judi Bar says, "Let's face it; most of us spend a large part of our workday sitting. Our bodies seem to adapt to sitting for long periods of time, and it's easy to stay glued to our chairs until we go home. But don't! Take the time to get up from your chair periodically. Not only does it invigorate your body and help you feel good, it also helps release muscle tension and gives you an extra boost of energy that can result in better concentration and more high-quality work."

Stand up

- Stand up: It does not matter how you stand up at first. Whether you lean on something—your knees, your chair—or not, keep doing it.

- Your ultimate goal is to be able to stand up without help, unsupported, without leaning forward but holding your head and back straight up.

- Start by using a hard-backed chair.

- Now, do that every 20–30 minutes when you are otherwise sitting at your desk, in a comfy chair with an electronic screen or book, or in front of the TV.

- At work, your productivity will go up while your physical health improves.

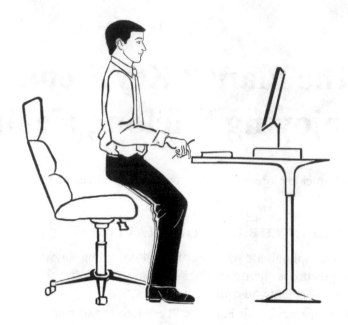

Figure 4. Correct posture for standing up.

- Stand up for a minute or so every 20–30 minutes during work. This could include walking to a restroom or getting water, but merely standing up without walking is fine. It is OK to move about but it is the change in posture signal that is crucial.

- Instead of texting your office colleagues, get up and visit them.

- Lift your arms up over your head, or you can walk slowly, or even do squats if you feel up to it. Practice standing up slowly, unsupported, and then sit down as slowly as you can.

- If you sit a lot, merely standing will have the single biggest impact on your risk factors for poor health and premature death.

Remember that the value of standing up is in the change of posture that tunes your body.

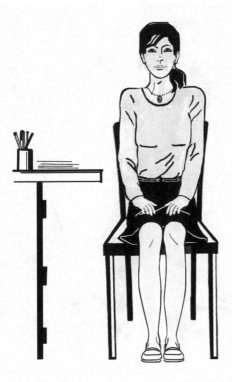

Figure 5. Correct posture for sitting up straight.

SIT UP

Sitting up is not as good as standing up, but it is as important. Gravity is just as important when sitting as while standing.

- Sitting with the head squarely supported by the neck and body, looking straight ahead, periodically sliding elbows back or stretching the arms to reach the ceiling, are all relieving moves that release tension, maintain good sitting posture, and tone core muscles.

- Sit at your desk with your screen at eye level when you are sitting up. Raise your sternum and show off your chest. If your chair has rollers, take them off or do not scoot around; get up instead.

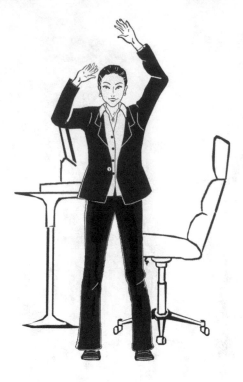

Figure 6. Stretching.

STRETCH UP

- Every time you stand up, stretch your arms up as high as you can. You may wave them over your head or stretch them gently to one side or the other.

- Even after the work day is over, continue to stand up every 20–30 minutes.

- Structure your day and evening to introduce necessary occasions to stand up (e.g. place your printer out of reach).

- Stand up during commercials if you are watching TV at home, or get up to get a drink, water your plants, cook, answer the door, when you are on the telephone, etc.

SIT DOWN

- Try to sit down as slowly as possible. The aim is eventually to be able to sit down slowly with your back straight and your head up over your spine.

- When using the toilet, try to sit down as slowly as you can without leaning on anything, just as when you stand up.

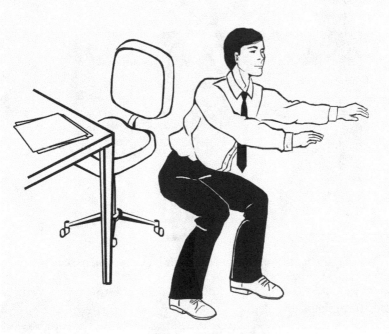

Figure 7. Squatting.

SQUAT OR KNEEL

Standing up from a full squat will increase the benefit of standing, giving you a longer gravity trajectory. Dr. Mercola, a leading osteopathic physician, suggests doing a squat to jump every 10 minutes for maximum gravity benefit. Equally lowering into a squat slowly will strengthen the posture-supporting muscles in your legs and back.

If you have Type II diabetes, Dr. Michael O. Thorner, Emeritus Professor of Endocrinology at the University of Virginia Department of Medicine, prescribes squatting three times every hour as the best activity treatment for his diabetic and pre-diabetic patients to control their blood sugar.

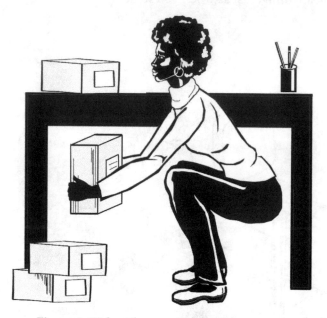

Figure 8. Pick up boxes with your legs, not your back.

- Squat to pick up a box instead of bending over—this spares your back and strengthens your legs.

- Relearn to squat while waiting in line—how far can you lower your seat, back straight, without bending your knees over your feet while raising your toes off the ground?

- Squat, kneel, or sit on the floor to play with a child.

- Think about how you sit and stand up when you use the toilet.

- Kneel often if squatting is difficult.

- Stand up from a squat or kneeling position until you can do it without support. That's what half the world population—at every age—does every day.

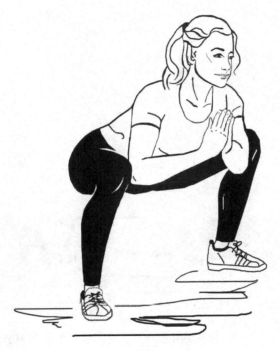

Figure 9. Sumo squat.

THE SUMO SQUAT

While speaking of squatting, let us not forget the sumo squat. At the Sedentary Behavior and Health Conference at the University of Illinois campus, in mid-October 2015, Dr. Neville Owen commented that he had not done his sumo squats that day. I had watched sumo wrestlers on TV, yet I had never thought of mimicking them, so I was intrigued by his comment. There and then in full view of everyone in the coffee shop he showed me how and I soon joined him. What a sight we must have been! But what a wonderful move it is that engages more muscles than I knew I had. I recommend it.

> "While 'cutting in' paint along a baseboard in a rather large living room, I came to the realization that simply getting up from a kneeling position, some 50 to 100 times a day, affected my overall health for the positive." —"Silvernail," comment on Movement Heals, YouTube.

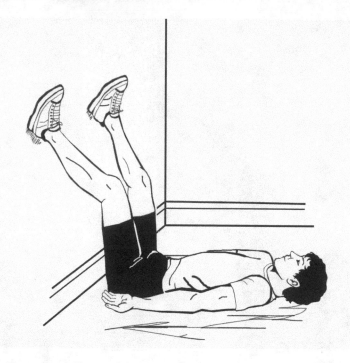

Figure 10. Lift your legs to improve blood flow throughout your body.

TURN UPSIDE-DOWN

- Stand on your head if you can, or try inversions.

- Challenge your head. Get your blood circulating to every part of the body.

- Hang onto monkey bars at the playground. Or lie on your stomach and hang your head down over the end of the bed to read.

- Lie on the floor with your legs in the air or leaning on a wall, or hang them over a couch with a pillow under your hips.

2. PAY ATTENTION TO YOUR POSTURE

Whether you are standing or sitting, pay attention to your posture. Whether you are sitting at your desk or are relaxing or texting your friends, it is important to maintain good posture. Avoid drooping your head forward or slouching your shoulders. It's bad for your neck and your

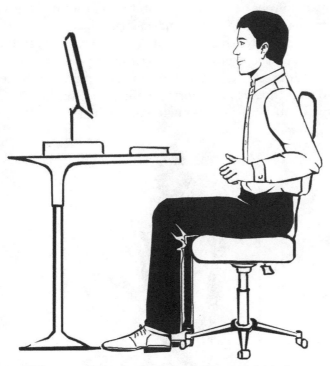

Figure 11. Slide your elbows back while sitting straight to improve posture.

spine. Sitting in a straight-backed chair instead of sinking into a soft comfy armchair or sofa makes keeping good posture easier. You can do stretches while sitting down the same as you do stretches standing up.

- Sit up. Raise your chest to the sky with shoulders pulled down. Stretch your arms up, palms clasped, fingers pointing up, hold your left wrist and pull your right hand up and to your left, keeping your right buttock firmly on the seat and your arms pulled back overhead. Can you feel the stretch up your right side? Hold it for one minute. Release slowly and repeat the stretch, pulling your left arm over with your right hand holding your left wrist.

- Roll your shoulders back to release any tension.

- Bend your arms. Slide your elbows back along your waist as far back as you can go. Do not bend your head. Hold for one minute and release.

- Holding onto your desk, slowly go back and forward doing a few cat-cows, rolling your head and shoulders forward, arching your back like a cat, feeling the stretch between your shoulder blades and reversing the motion, chest and head up with arms stretched, feeling the stretch around your chest and back. With shoulders pulled down, lean your head to your shoulder, chin forward, then, keeping your head in that position, rotate your chin gently to your shoulder. Feel the stretch in

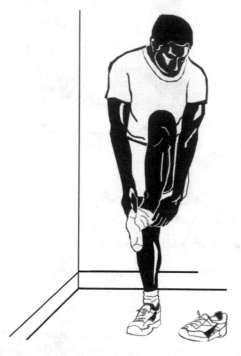

Figure 12. Dressing and undressing standing up will improve your balance and coordination.

your neck.

3. REINFORCE YOUR BALANCE AND COORDINATION MAPS

- Stimulate the proprioceptors (balance sensors) in your feet and in your seat.

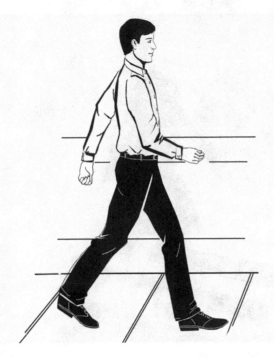

Figure 13. Hold your head up and your back straight while walking.

- Dress and undress while standing up. Start out by leaning on the wall or the bed. Within a couple of weeks, you will be able to put your pants on, and even socks or pantyhose, standing up if you keep at it.

- When you walk, hold your head up and your shoulders back.

- While waiting in queue at the post office or check-out counter, stand up straight, what yogis call mountain pose, with your head well balanced over your spine and your chest raised up, shoulders back. Then stand momentarily with your weight on only one leg at a time.

- Even if you are sitting, sit up straight or put a book on your head. You will need to maintain correct posture if you want to keep that book up there.

- Dance! Even when you are home by yourself!

- Paint a wall. Start with a low step stool and move up as you feel more confident.

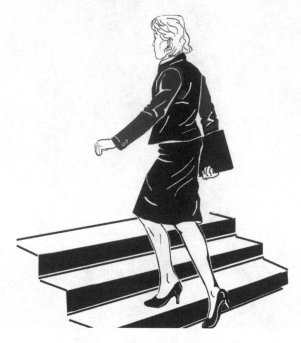

Figure 14. Whenever possible, take the stairs instead of the elevator.

- Go up and down the stairs, holding the railing at first until you can do without it.

- Stand on one leg as long as you can and then the other. Time yourself. When you master it, try it with your eyes shut.

- Keep up your walking habit.

You think of walking as a milder form of aerobic exercise, and so it is, but just as doing housework and gardening, walking can expend a lot of calories as well. If you view taking a walk with friends as your daily exercise requirement, you may make the mistake of considering that you have fulfilled your daily moving requirement. Walking is the most comprehensive balance and coordination movement. Therefore, you need to do it often to maintain strong legs and a balanced stepping motion, both sideways and moving forward. But as in all other movement, you need to do it correctly: use upright posture, swing your arms, aim to take steps with your feet closer to each other, and eventually use naturally longer strides. As we age (or in astronauts returning from a space mission), we tend to stand with feet wider

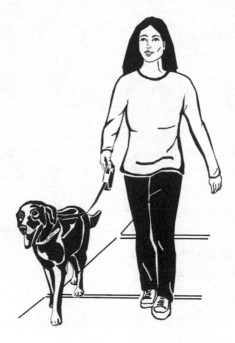

Figure 15. Walk your dog more. Your dog will love you for it.

apart for stability and our steps are shorter. We also tend to hang our head down, looking at our feet. You may want to try walking with your arms crossed behind your back, clasping as near to your elbows as you can get them and pushing your chest up, with your eyes looking straight ahead. Letting your eyes look down at your feet for safety will encourage stooping, which can be detrimental to your health. Walking is the best exercise for coordination of movement and all-around balance. In addition, it affects how you feel. And your mood can affect how you walk. If you are sad, your shoulders are slumped, whereas if you are happy, you find yourself bouncing along. Johannes Rhode and his colleagues at the Canadian Institute for Advanced Research found that it works the other way as well. How you walk affects your mood. So putting a spring in your walk or sharing a happy conversation with walking partners contributes to positive feelings.

> "Walk at moderate intensity or 100 steps per minute, hum or listen to the Bee Gees' song 'Staying Alive' while you walk. The song's tempo is 100 beats per minute," says Simon Marshall, Ph.D. at U.C. San Diego.

4. Smart moving

Seek out chances to move more and in different ways—it's a self-fulfilling prophecy. *There are virtually unlimited opportunities for movement throughout the day.*

Here are some ideas to choose from—you'll figure out the ones that work for you, your lifestyle, and your physical abilities:

- Take the stairs whenever possible instead of the elevator or escalator. As with standing and sitting, you use different muscles in the back of your legs to step down. Hold the railing at first for safety but aim not to use it to pull yourself up.

- Park as far as possible from your work or destination, or take public transport, to build moving into your day. Carry your groceries.

- Walk your dog more. It's the chore that isn't.

- Cook meals or soups from scratch. Bonus here is better nutrition and tastier food.

- Plant a garden. Gardening is a wonderful activity that gets you into nature, even if it's 10 feet from your home.

- Resolve to do more to clean and maintain your home and car. Healthier you, nicer home and car.

- Replace one car trip a week with human power. Walk or bike or use public transport. Just being outside is so wonderful.

- See your best friends during a walk or hike, or in the garden, instead of over a meal or sitting in front of the TV.

- Play a sport as long as you can—tennis, table tennis, golf, or mini-golf.

- Dance.

Esther, a resident at Leisure World, came to one of my talks with a walker. When asked about exercise, she said "I dance! I turn up the music loud and use my kitchen chairs, which are on rollers, and I dance around the kitchen and sing!"

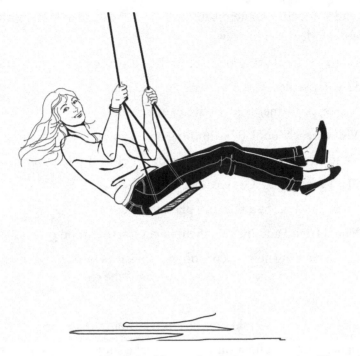

Figure 16. Swinging provides valuable gravity-resistant exercise. No one has to know that you're having fun, too.

5. GET UP AND PLAY!

As we age, we tend to stop playing. Ever notice how most of us were a bit thinner when we were young? Pledge to reverse that and play!

Dr. Stephen Jepson, a leading potter and ceramics professor at a Florida university, turned to developing the art of playing in his 70s as a means of maintaining youth. He is now an outstanding speaker around the world, travelling with his Never Leave the Playground program, teaching, demonstrating, and entertaining audiences. If you wonder how you can possibly begin playing again, he recommends to try juggling. Use a few tennis balls at first to get the hang of it and go from there—it's a great way to make friends with young and old and regain your balance in the process. Dr. John Kitchin, a retired neuropsychiatrist, does it a different way. Also in his 70s, he took up roller-blading along Marina del Ray in LA, making lots of new friends along the way, while recognizing the value of fun and using gravity and keeping up his sense of balance as a bonus.

Spend some time contemplating what you really enjoy doing and do it. Need an idea? Here's a few:

- Go to the local playground or park and swing on a swing. Gravity +!
- Play hopscotch. Great for strength and balance.
- Dance! A partner is nice but not essential.
- Visit a beach, pool, or swimming hole and get wet with some friends.
- Go to an amusement park and enjoy the rides. Roller coasters are great.
- Make something. Get creative. Paint, decorate.
- Take your bike to a safe, fun place to ride.
- Find a friend and include them in your activity and games.
- Try something new like paddling a sea kayak or playing a game of golf. Even miniature golf will keep you out of the chair.
- Try juggling.
- Play tennis or golf, ski or surf. Pole ski walk in the park.
- In the winter, build a snowman or make snow angels. Or for the more fit, go cross country or downhill skiing with friends and family. You don't have to go fast or hard.
- Skip a rope, do jumping jacks, crouch, and jump (that can be up to 6G), jump on a trampoline (about 4.5G). Increase your gravity stimulus intermittently on a centrifuge (if you can find one), ride a roller coaster, hypervibe, or gyrogym. They all amplify the gravity stimulus.

6. SEEK ANCIENT PRACTICES

Yoga, tai chi, quijong, the Alexander Technique—take a few classes or practice at home. Any or all of these rely on moving in gravity and mimic movements in nature observed in trees, plants, birds, and animals.

A 20-minute bout of yoga was found to stimulate memory and brain function better than 20 minutes of running on a treadmill. The practice of yoga is about moving naturally, not exercising. It is called a practice because, simply put, you practice moving.

The Alexander Technique is another method that incorporates much of yoga and tai chi so that you learn *how to move* when you do anything that

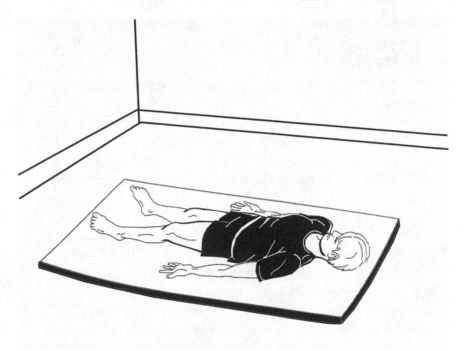

Figure 17. Relaxation.

involves "moving," like walking, running, sitting, lifting, eating, knitting, golfing, swimming, sweeping, and so on. You learn where you are over-tensing or over-contracting your muscles and therefore your joints, which creates stiffness and pain.

7. RELAXATION

Your body needs to relax totally in order to get the most out of movement. Otherwise, the movement is only a part of what it can be.

- Our muscles are at least partially contracted all the time to support us upright. Total relaxation requires consciously letting go, giving in to gravity.
- Lying on the floor or in water provides ultimate relaxation.
- Slowing down breathing, consciously slowing one's heart rate, lowering blood pressure, and clearing one's mind all help you achieve invigorating total relaxation.

- Mind/body practices help you become more aware (so that you truly notice how you feel and then can take more effective, safe actions), while the body benefits from slow, gravity-using activities.

- Practice body scanning. This simple mindfulness meditation focuses on breathing. As you scan your body, you realize the process reduces your heart rate and blood pressure and relaxes your muscles, skin, tendons, ligaments, and organs.

Smart moving is natural moving, but it requires your conscious participation. The key to its success is for it to become second nature, a habit, just as it once was!

The more you move, the more you will want to move. Notice how children start to fidget restlessly if you make them sit still. The more you move, the more your body will tell you when it needs to move again.

Moving becomes naturally energizing, a virtuous cycle. It will leave you feeling better throughout the day.

The benefits of natural, non-strenuous, frequent daily smart movement will mean a healthier, happier, more mobile and productive you, today as well as later in your life.

8. Look inward and change your habits

From the moment you wake up to the time you shut your eyes to sleep become aware of the following:

- Where you are
- What are you doing
- How you feel
- Be ready to make adjustments:
  - Check your attitude
  - Make new moving habits

Takeaway messages

Embrace these no sweat, natural smart moves to feel good:

- Stoke up on energy all day long
- Gain precious time by dropping your exercise addiction

- Household chores add money to your pocket
- Regain your balance
- Lose your aches and pains and stiff neck
- Being happy is child's play *and* adult's play
- Lose weight without trying every time you stand up
- Give in to gravity and stay young and healthy
- Keep up your walking habit
- Make a habit of moving
- Love living

The bottom line is that by staying active, moving, and connected, you gain the reward of having energy all day, sleeping well at night, and feeling healthy, happy, and fulfilled.

Just remember—your body is designed to move.

Acknowledgments

I never thought I would be writing another book about how bad sitting is for you. But the subject clearly has not died, nor has it been solved so many years later. In fact, the problem is worse than ever. Public interest has grown. We are sitting more than ever. An industry of technological solutions is growing. That's when Kent Sorsky asked if "there was another book in me"! So I have to thank Kent for the stimulus to put pen to paper as well as my son George for his support throughout, working assiduously while drafting a short guide on the most effective ways to move that was incorporated in this book. My wonderful husband patiently copyedited numerous versions. Two outstanding conferences of the best in the business also happened during this period of waiting—first the Sedentary Behavior and Health conference in Urbana, Illinois, was chaired by professors Neville Owen and Weimo Zhou; the second at the Ergonomics Conference in Las Vegas was chaired by professor Alan Hedge. An invited lecture at the prestigious Institute for Human and Machine Cognition in Pensacola, Florida, followed. These conferences gave me the opportunity to air my views and sharpen my perspective. I am deeply indebted to all who attended for their questions and positive feedback.

Then came the hard part of putting it all together. Fortunately, my wonderful editor Elsa Peterson came to the rescue. She is a magician at making sense and putting order to my story. I am forever grateful.

Needless to say that as in the past, my gratitude and respect go to the remarkable men and women, American and Russian, who volunteered to be test subjects in space or in ground studies. Their contribution will help others stay healthy on their way to Mars or live long and healthy lives back here on earth. Every day and with every space flight mission we gain greater appreciation of how gravity interacts with the human body. We have just broken the six-month duration in space for the United States with the record-making flight of Scott Kelly. It's only just begun.

Endnotes

1. Vernikos, J. "Space and Aging: Parallel Processes." NASA pamphlet, 1986.

2. Sandler H., Vernikos J. (eds.,) *Inactivity: Its Physiology*. New York: Academic Press, 1986.

3. Vernikos, J. *The G-Connection: Harness Gravity and Reverse Aging*. iUniverse, 2004.

4. Ekelund, U., Steene-Johanessen, J., Brown W.J., Fagerland, M.W., Owen, N., Powell, K.E., Bauman, A., Lee, I-Min. "Physical activity attenuates the detrimental association of sitting time with mortality: A harmonised meta-analysis of data from more than one million men and women." *Lancet* (July, 2016): DOI: 10.1016/S0140-6736(16)30370-1.

5. Dunlap, D., Song, J., Arnston, E., Semanik, P., Lee, J., Chang, R., Hootman, J.M. "Sedentary time in US older adults associated with disability in activities of daily living independent of physical activity." *Journal of Physical Activity & Health* (2015): 12(3):93-101.

6. Levine, A.J. *Get Up! Why Your Chair Is Killing You and What You Can Do About It*. New York: Palgrave Macmillan, 2014, p. 234.

7. Hamilton, M.T., Hamilton, D.G., Zderic, T.W. "Role of low energy expenditure and sitting in obesity, metabolic syndrome, type-2 diabetes and cardiovascular disease." *Diabetes* (2007): 56(11):2655–2667.

8. Hamilton, M.T., Hamilton, D.G., Zderic, T.W., Owen, N. "Too Little Exercise and Too Much Sitting: Inactivity Physiology and the Need for New Recommendations on Sedentary Behavior." *Curr Cardiovasc Risk Rep.* (July 2008): 2(4):292–298.

9. Vernikos, J., Ludwig, D.A., Ertl, A.C., Wade, C.E., Keil, L.C., O'Harra, D. "Effect of Standing or Walking on Physiological Changes Induced by Head-Down Bed Rest." *Aviat Space Env Med* (1996): 67:1069–1079

10. Engelke, K.A., Doerr, D.F., Convertino, V.A. "A single bout of exhaustive exercise affects integrated baroreflex function after 16 days of head-down tilt." *American Journal of Physiology* (1995): 269:R614–620.

11. Lynch, B.M., Neville, Owen. "Too Much Sitting and Chronic Disease Risk: Steps to Move the Science Forward." *Ann of Int Med* (2015): 162:146–147.

12. American Heart Association (statistics on sedentary jobs and average work week): http://www.heart.org/HEARTORG/GettingHealthy/PhysicalActivity/FitnessBasics/The-Price-of-Inactivity_UCM_307974_Article.jsp#

13. Lewis, S., Hennekens, C. "Regular Physical Activity: Forgotten Benefits." *Amer J Med* (2016): 129(2):137-138.

14. Wilmot, E.G., Edwardson, C.L., Achana, F.A., Davies, M.J., Gorely, T., Gray, L.J., Khunti, K., Yates, T., Biddle, S.J.H. "Sedentary Time in Adults and the Association with Diabetes, Cardiovascular Disease and Death: Systematic Review and Meta-Analysis." *Diabetologia* (2012): 55(11):2895–2905.

15. Virtanen, M., Heikkila, K., Jokela, M., Ferrie, J.E., Batty, G.D., Vahtera, J., Kimivaki, M. " Long Working Hours and Coronary Heart Disease: A Systematic Review and Meta-Analysis." *Amer J Epidemiol* (2012): 176 (7): 586-596.

16. Veerman, J.L., Healy, G.N., Cobiac, L.J., Vos, T., Winkler, E.A.H., Owen, N., Dunstan, D.W. "Television Viewing Time and Reduced Life Expectancy: A Life Table Analysis." *Br J Sports Med* (2012): 46:927–930.

17. Katzmarzyk, P.T., Church, T.S., Craig, C.L., Bouchard, C. "Sitting Time and Mortality from All Causes, Cardiovascular Disease and Cancer." *Med Sci Sports Ex* (2009): 41:998–1005.

18. Matthews, C.E., Bowles, H.R., Blair, A., Park, Y., Troiano, R.P., Hollenbeck, A., Schatzkin, A. "Amount of Time Spent in Sedentary Behaviors and Cause-Specific Mortality in U.S. Adults." *Am J ClinNutr* (2012): 96:437–445.

19. Dunstan, D.W., Kingwell, B.A., Larsen, R., Healy, G.N., Cerin, E., Hamilton, M.T., Shaw, J.E., Bertovic, D.A., Zimmet, P.Z., Salmon, J., Owen, N. "Breaking Up Prolonged Sitting Reduces Postprandial Glucose and Insulin Responses." *Diabetes Care* (2012): 35 (5):976–983.doi:10.2337/dc11–1931.

20. Lynch, B.M. "Sedentary Behavior and Cancer: A Systematic Review of the Literature and Proposed Biological Mechanisms." *Cancer Epid Biomarkers Prev* (2007): 19:2691–2709.

21. Schmid, D., Leitzman, M.F. "Sedentary Behavior Increases the Risk of Certain Cancers." *JNCI* (2014): 106(7):dju206.

22. Kulinski, J. "Sedentary Behavior Is Associated with Coronary Artery Calcification." Abstract from the Dallas Heart Study, 64th Annual Meeting of the American College of Cardiology, San Diego, CA.

23. Saurabh, S.T., Bielko, S.L., Mather, K.J., Johnston, J.D., Wallace, J.P. "Effect of Prolonged Sitting and Breaks in Sitting Time on Endothelial Function." *Medicine & Science in Sports and Exercise* (2015): 47:843-849.

24. Rohme Young, D., Reynolds, K., Sidell, M., Brar, S., Ghai, N.R., Sternfeld, B., Jacosen, S.J., Slezac, J.M., Caan, B., Quinn, V.P. "Effects of Physical Activity and Sedentary Time on the Risk of Heart Failure." *Circulation: Heart Failure* (2014): 7:21-27.

25. Saunders, T.J., Larouche, R., Colley, R.C., Tremblay, M.S. "Acute Sedentary Behaviour and Markers of Cardiometabolic Risk: A Systematic Review of Intervention Studies." *Journal of Nutrition and Metabolism* (2012): (4): 712435, 12 pp.

26. Ekelund, U., et al. "Physical Activity and All-cause Mortality Across Levels of Overall and Abdominal Adiposity in European Men and Women: the European Perspective Investigation into Cancer and Nutrition Study (EPIC)" *American Journal of Clinical Nutrition* (2015): 101(3): 613-621.

27. Bey, L., Hamilton, M.T. "Suppression of Skeletal Muscle Lipoprotein Lipase Activity During Physical Inactivity: A Molecular Reason to Maintain Daily Low Intensity Activity." *J. Physiol* (2003): 551:673–682.

28. Neuhaus, M., Healy, G.N., Dunstan, D.W., Owen, N., Eakin, E.G. "Workplace Sitting and Height-Adjustable Workstations: A Randomized Controlled Trial." *Am J Prev Med* (2014): 46:30–40. doi: 10.1016/j.amepre.2013.09.009.

29. Bergouignan, A., Rudwill, F., Simon, C., Blanc, S.. "Physical Inactivity as the Culprit of Metabolic Inflexibility: Evidence from Bed-Rest Studies." *J Appl Physiol* (2011): 111:1201–1210.

30. Sloan, R.A., Sawada, S., Susumu, S., Girdano, D., Liu, Tong, Liu, Yi, Biddle, S.J.H., Blair, S.N. "Associations of Sedentary Behavior and Physical Activity with Psychological Distress: A Cross-Sectional Study from Singapore." *BMC Public Health* (2013): 13(1):885.

31. Andrews, L.W. *Psychology Today* (March, 2014): Three year survey of 25,000 workers concluded mental health damaged. Lead author Tetsuya Nakazawa, of Chiba University in Japan.

32. Nakazawa, T. "Too Much Computer Work Causes Insomnia and Depression." *Amer J Industr Med* (2003).

33. Aaltonen, S., Latvala, A., Rose, R.J., Pulkkinen, L. ,Kujala, U.M., Kaprio, J., Silvetoinen, K. "Motor Development and Physical Activity: A Longitudinal Discordant Twin-Pair Study." *Med Sci Sports Ex* (2015): 47:(10):2111-2118.

34. Li, K., Guo, X., Jin, Z., Ouyang, X., Zeng, Y., Feng J., Wang, Y., Ma, L. "Effect of Simulated Microgravity on Human Brain Gray Matter and White Matter—Evidence from MRI." *PLOS ONE* (Aug., 2015): 13:10(8):e013583.

35. Burzynska, A. "Sedentary Behavior May Counteract Brain Benefits of Exercise in Older Adults." *PLOS ONE.* (Sept., 2014).

36. De Boer, M.D. "Viewing as Little as 1 Hour of Television Daily Is Associated with Higher Weight Status in Kindergartners: The Early Childhood Longitudinal Study." American Academy of Pediatrics Mtg, San Diego, CA, April 26th, 2015.

37. Strauss, Valerie. "Why-so-many-kids-cant-sit-still-in-school-today." *Washington Post* (July 8th, 2014): https://www.washingtonpost.com/news/ answer-sheet/ wp/2014/07/08/why-so-many-kids-cant-sit-still-in-schooltoday/

38. Dentro, K.N., Beals, K., Crouter, S.E., et al. Results from the United States' 2014 Report Card on Physical Activity for Children and Youth, *Journal of Physical Activity and Health* (2014): 11 (Supplement 1), S105–S112.

39. Harvard School of Public Health, 2013, report on children and weight: http://www. rwjf.org/en/library/research/2013/02/a-poll-about-children-and-weight.html.

40. Mehta, R.K., Shortz, A.E., Benden, M.E. "StandingUp for Learning: A Pilot Investigation on Neurocognitive Benefits of Stand-Biased School Desks." *International J Env Res & Pub Health* (2015): 13:(0059)DOI: 10.3390/ ijerph13010059.

41. Chari, R., Warsh, J., Ketterer, T., Hossain, J., Shariff, I. "Association Between Health Literacy and Child and Adolescent Obesity." *Patient Educ Couns* (2014) 94(1):61-644.

42. Chaddock-Heyman, L., Hillman, C.H., Cohen, N.J., Kramer III, A.F. "The Importance of Physical Activity and Aerobic Fitness for Cognitive Control and Memory in Children." *Monographs of the Society for Research in Child Development* (2014): 79: 255.

43. Myers, G.D., Faigenbaum, A.D., Edwards, N.M., Clark, J.F., Best, T.M., Sallis, R.E. "Sixty Minutes of What? A Developing Brain Perspective for Activating Children with an Integrative Exercise Approach." *Br J Sports Med.* (Mar, 2015): 49(5):282-9.

44. Peper, E., Lin, I-Mei. "Increase or Decrease Depression: How Body Postures Influence Your Energy Level." *Biofeedback* (2012): 40:(3) 125-130.546.

45. Carr, L.J., Leonhard, C., Tucker, S., Fethke, N., Benzo, R., Gerr, F. "Total Worker Health Intervention Increases Activity of Sedentary Workers." *American Journal of Preventive Medicine* (2015): DOI: 10.1016/j.amepre.2015.06.022.

46. Rosenkrantz, S.K., Mailey, E.L. "Sitting Time Associated with Increased Risk of Chronic Disease." *Int J. Behav Nutr & Phys Act* (2013). Also, "Experts Offer Little Tips to Make Big Changes in Work Health." *MedicalxPress.com* (June 24, 2015).

47. Seguin, R., Buchner, D.M., Liu, J., Allison, M., Manini, T., Wang, C-Y, Manson, J.E., Messina, C.R., Patel, M.J., Moreland, L., Stefanik, M.L., LaCroix, A.Z. "Sedentary Behavior and Mortality in Older Women, The Women's Health Initiative." *Amer.J. Prev Med.* (Feb, 2014): 46: 122-135.

48.   http://www.theonion.com/articles/health-experts-recommendstanding-up-at-deskleavi,379

49. Leupker, R., quoted in an interview with *Medpage Today* (2014): "Anything that gets people up and moving around is probably a good thing . . . People don't move enough in work time or leisure time . . . Our entire culture has become more sedentary. Physical activity has been engineered out of people's lives."

50. Barzilai, N., Huffman, D.M., Muzumdar, R.H., Bartke, A. "The Critical Role of Metabolic Pathways in Aging." *Diabetes* (2012): 61(6):1315–1322. doi: 10.2337/db111300.

51. Hupin, D., Roche, F., Gremeaux, V., Chatard, J.C., Oriol, M., Gaspoz, J.M. Barthelemy, J.C., Edouard, P. "Even a Low-Dose of Moderate-to-Vigorous Physical Activity Reduces Mortality by 22% in Adults Aged ≥60 Years: A Systematic Review and Meta-Analysis." *Br J Sports Med* (2015): 49:1262-1267.

52. Sardinha, L.B., Santos, D.A., Silva, A.M., Baptista, F., Owen, N. "Breaking-up Sedentary Time Is Associated with Physical Function in Older Adults." *J Gerontol A Biol Sci Med Sci* (2014.): doi: 10.1093/Gerona/glu1933.

53. Blackburn, E., Epel, E.S., Lin, J. "Human Telomere Biology: A Contributory and Interactive Factor in Aging, Disease Risks, and Protection." *Science* (2015): 35996265): 1193-1198.

54. Collins, M., Renault, V., Grobler, L.A., et al. "Athletes with Exercise-Associated Fatigue Have Abnormally Short Muscle DNA Telomeres." *Med Sci Sports Ex* (2003): 35(9):1524–8.

55. Cherkas, L.F., Hunkin, J.L., Kato, B.S., Richards, J.B., Gardner, J.P., Surdulescu, G.L., Kimura, M., Lu, X., Spector, T.D., Aviv, A. "The Association between Physical Activity in Leisure Time and Leukocyte Telomere Length." *Arch Intern Med* (2008): 168(2):154–8.

56. Ludlow, A.T., Zimmerman, J.B., Witkowski, S., Hearn, J.W., Hatfield, B., Roth, S.M. "Relationship between Physical Activity Level, Telomere Length, and Telomerase Activity." *Med Sci Sports Ex* (2008): 40(10): 1764–1771. doi:10.1249/MSS.0b013e31817c92aa.

57. Benden, M.E., Blake, J.J., Wendel, M.L., Huber Jr., J.C. "The Impact of Stand-Biased Desks in Classrooms on Calorie Expenditure in Children." *American Journal Public Health* (2011): 101 (8).

58. Saurabh ST, Bielko SL, Mather KJ, Johnston JD, Wallace JP. 2015. "Effect of Prolonged Sitting and Breaks in Sitting Time on Endothelial Function." *Medicine & Science in Sports and Exercise* 47:843-849

59. Nielsen, R.O., Schierling, P., Tesch, P., Stat, P., Langsberg, H. "Collagen Content in the Vastus Lateralis and Soleus Muscle Following a 90-Day Bed-Rest Period With or Without Resistance Exercises." *Muscles Ligaments Tendons J* (2016): 5(4):305–309. Doi: 10.11138/mlti/2015.5.4.305.

60. Barone Gibbs, B., Gabriel, K.P., Reis, J.P., Jakicic, J.M., Carbethon, M.R., Sternfeld, B. "Cross-Sectional and Longitudinal Associations Between Objectively Measured Sedentary Time and Metabolic Disease: The Coronary Artery Risk Development in Young Adults (CARDIA) Study." *Diabetes Care* (2015): doi: 10.2337/dc15-0226 July 8, 2015.

61. Falconer, C.L., Andrews, A.C., Cooper, R.C., Ashley, R. "The Potential of Displacing Sedentary Time in Adults with Type 2 Diabetes." *Med in Sports & Exercise* (March, 2015): doi: 10. 1249/MSS.000000000000651.

62. Henson, J., Yates, T., Biddle, S.J.H., Edwardson, C.L., Khunti, K. "Associations of Objectively Measuring Sedentary Behaviour and Physical Activity with Markers of Cardiometabolic Health." *Diabetologia* (2013):·DOI:1007/s00125-013-2845-9.

63. Eddie, Phillips, quoted in "Interrupting Sitting Time May Improve Health in Type 2 Diabetes." March 26, 2015, www.Foxnews.com.

64. Luder, R. "Chairs Ergonomics," National Ergonomics Conference & Ergo Expo, Las Vegas (2015).

65. Congleton, J.J. "Maximizing Your Ergonomic and Safety Program with Lean Concepts," National Ergonomics Conference & Ergo Expo Las Vegas (2016).

66. Anshell, J. *Smart Medicine for Your Eyes: A Guide to Natural, Effective, and Safe Relief of Common Eye Disorders.* New York: Square One, 2015.

67. Gokhale, E. *8 Steps to a Pain-Free Back.* Pendo Press, 2008.

68. Huang, Li, Galinsky, A. "Mind–Body Dissonance: Conflict Between the Senses Expands the Mind's Horizons." *Social Psych & Personality Science*, (2011) 2(4): 351-359.

69. Cuddy, A, "Your Body Language Shapes Who You Are." TED Talks (2012): http://www.ted.com/talks/amy_cuddy_your_body_language_shapes_who_you_are

Index

ABOUT THE AUTHOR

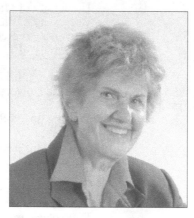

JOAN VERNIKOS, PH.D., is a pioneering medical research scientist who has conducted seminal studies in space medicine, inactivity physiology, stress, and healthy aging. Born in Alexandria, Egypt, in 1934, Vernikos received her Ph.D. in pharmacology at the University of London and became a researcher at the NASA Ames Research Center in 1964. She was a foundational figure of space medicine research and served as Life Sciences Director at the NASA Ames Research Center from 1986 to 1993 and Director of the Life Sciences Division at NASA headquarters from 1993 to 2000.

In her research at NASA, Vernikos spearheaded groundbreaking medical studies on the effects of weightlessness on health. Vernikos' NASA research on the health effects of weightlessness helped establish the scientific causal relationship between sedentary living, rapid aging, and poor health.

Vernikos has been twice winner of NASA's Exceptional Leadership Award, and she has also received NASA's Exceptional Scientific Achievement Award, the Melbourne Boynton Award from the American Astronautical Association, the Strughold Award in Space Medicine from the American Aerospace Medical Association, the Jeffries Award from the American Institute of Aeronautics and Astronautics, the Lifetime Achievement Award from Women in Aerospace, and numerous other academic and scientific awards.

Vernikos has written four previous books: *Inactivity: Physiological Effects* (1987, co-written with Harold Sandler), *The G-Connection: Harness Gravity and Reverse Aging* (2004), *Stress Fitness for Seniors* (2009), and *Sitting Kills, Moving Heals* (2011).

Books for the Best Half of Life from Quill Driver Books

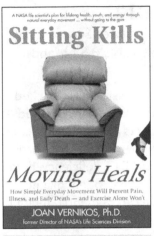

$14.95 ($16.95 Canada)

Sitting Kills, Moving Heals

How Simple Everyday Movement Will Prevent Pain, Illness, and Early Death—and Exercise Alone Won't

by Joan Vernikos, Ph.D., former Director of NASA's Life Sciences Division

New medical research has shown that sitting too much will shorten your life, even if you get regular exercise. *Sitting Kills, Moving Heals* shows that the key to lifelong fitness and good health is constant, nonstrenuous movement that resists the force of gravity. This easy-to-follow, common-sense plan will show you how simple, everyday, and fun activities like walking, gardening, dancing, golf, and more will keep you fit, strong and independent your whole life long.

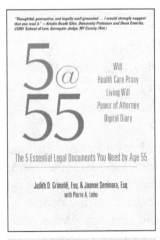

$12.95 ($13.95 Canada)

5@55

The 5 Essential Legal Documents You Need by Age 55

by Judith D. Grimaldi, Esq. & Joanne Seminara, Esq. with Pierre A. Lehu

Written by experienced elder law attorneys, *5@55* is a slim, easy-to-read guide to the five most important legal documents you should have by age 55. *5@55* explains in plain English why these documents are necessary, what legal issues you need to be aware of, what pitfalls to avoid and how to work with your lawyer to make sure that your decisions will be followed. An easy and reassuring guide to making important legal decisions, *5@55* is a must-have manual for the second half of life.

Available from bookstores, online bookstores, and QuillDriverBooks.com, or by calling toll-free 1-800-345-4447.

Protect your family's health with Quill Driver Books

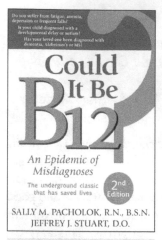

$14.95 ($16.95 Canada)

Could It Be B12?

An Epidemic of Misdiagnoses Second Edition
by Sally M. Pacholok, R.N., B.S.N., and
Jeffrey J. Stuart, D.O.

The underground classic that sparked a patients' rebellion and saved lives! *Could It Be B12?* reveals the facts about a health crisis most doctors don't know exists—the chronic misdiagnosis of vitamin B12 deficiency. If you or your loved ones have been diagnosed with Alzheimer's disease, dementia, multiple sclerosis, depression, fatigue, mental illness, frequent falls, forgetfulness, or other disorders, B12 deficiency may be the underlying cause. *Could It Be B12?* gives you the knowledge to take control of your health.

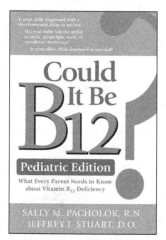

$16.95 ($22.95 Canada)

Could It Be B12? Pediatric Edition

What Every Parent Needs to Know About Vitamin B12 Deficiency
by Sally M. Pacholok, R.N., and
Jeffrey J. Stuart, D.O.

Written by the authors of the acclaimed *Could It Be B12?*, *Could It Be B12? Pediatric Edition* offers parents necessary information about protecting children from B12 deficiency from fetal development through adolescence. Presenting strategies to detect, prevent, and treat B12 deficiency–caused disorders, *Could It Be B12? Pediatric Edition* is a must-read for all parents, expectant parents, teachers, and healthcare providers.

Available from bookstores, online bookstores, and
QuillDriverBooks.com, or by calling toll-free 1-800-345-4447.

CPSIA information can be obtained
at www.ICGtesting.com
Printed in the USA
JSHW041709020222
22513JS00008B/175